IMPLANT PROSTHODONTICS
CLINICAL AND LABORATORY PROCEDURES

IMPLANT PROSTHODONTICS

CLINICAL AND LABORATORY PROCEDURES

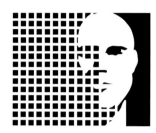

EDWARD J. FREDRICKSON, D.D.S., F.I.C.D.

Private Practice, Prosthodontics,
Spokane, Washington

PATRICK J. STEVENS, D.D.S

Private Practice, Prosthodontics,
Spokane, Washington

MAURICE L. GRESS, C.D.T., F.N.B.C.

President, AU Dental Ceramics, Inc.,
Spokane, Washington

with 609 *illustrations, including* 585 *in color*

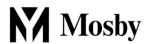 **Mosby**

St. Louis Baltimore Berlin Boston Carlsbad Chicago London Madrid
Naples New York Philadelphia Sydney Tokyo Toronto

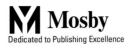

Mosby
Dedicated to Publishing Excellence

Publisher: George Stamathis
Editor-in-Chief: Don Ladig
Executive Editor: Linda L. Duncan
Developmental Editor: Melba Steube
Project Manager: Patricia Tannian
Production Editor: Barbara Jeanne Wilson
Senior Book Designer: Gail Morey Hudson
Manufacturing Supervisor: Karen Lewis
Cover Designer: Teresa Breckwoldt

Printed in the United States of America
Composition by Graphic World, Inc./Accu-Color, Inc.
Printing/binding by Walsworth Publishing Co.

Mosby–Year Book, Inc.
11830 Westline Industrial Drive
St. Louis, Missouri 63146

Library of Congress Cataloging in Publication Data
Fredrickson, Edward J.
    Implant prosthodontics : clinical and laboratory procedures /
Edward J. Fredrickson, Patrick J. Stevens, Maurice L. Gress.
      p.   cm.
    Includes bibliographical references and index.
    ISBN 0-8016-1635-2
    1. Osseointegrated dental implants. I. Stevens, Patrick J.
II. Gress, Maurice L. III. Title.
    [DNLM: 1. Dental Implants. 2. Dental Prosthesis—methods.
3. Dental Implantation, Endosseous—methods. WU 640 F852i 1994]
RK667.I45F74   1994
617.6'9—dc20
DNLM/DLC
for Library of Congress   93-46993
                                                      CIP

94 95 96 97 98 / 9 8 7 6 5 4 3 2 1

Contributors

KENJI W. HIGUCHI, D.D.S, M.S.

Private Practice,
Spokane, Washington

GAYLE S. ORTON, R.D.H., B.S., M.Ed.

Associate Professor and Chairperson,
Department of Dental Hygiene,
Eastern Washington University,
Spokane, Washington

DEBORAH LYNN STEELE, R.D.H., B.S.

Adjunct Faculty,
Department of Dental Hygiene,
Eastern Washington University;
Registered Dental Hygienist,
Spokane Center for Implant Prosthodontics,
Spokane, Washington

Foreword

Rehabilitation of the edentulous patient relies on safe and lasting retention of a prosthesis that provides adequate anatomical and functional restitution.

Each patient must receive an individual therapeutic solution, whichever technical modality (crown bridge or overdenture) is preferred.

This book is an important guide to correct clinical handling of prosthetic procedures in osseointegrated reconstruction and is based on the authors' own experiences and observations.

Per-Ingvar Branemark

Professor, M.D., Ph.D., O.Dhc.

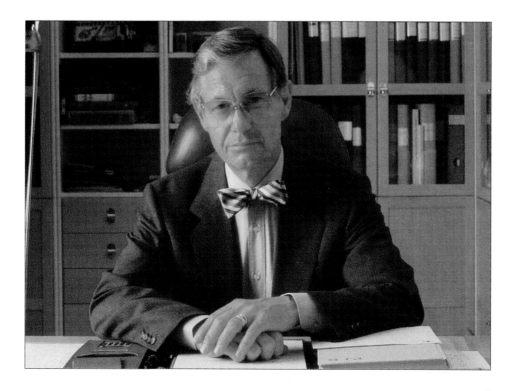

Foreword

Dr. Edward J. Fredrickson represents the epitome of the private sector in the practice of prosthetic dentistry. He and his carefully chosen colleagues, Dr. Patrick J. Stevens and Mr. Maurice L. Gress, C.D.T., F.N.B.C., have written a landmark text, which represents the culmination of accumulated knowledge, experience, and skill in the clinical and laboratory treatment of patients with dental implants. Dental implants have been a component of the armamentarium of the practicing dentist for over 40 years.

The current recognition of dental implant therapy as an acceptable clinical modality is directly due to the principles, concepts, and practices of the Branemark system as developed and promulgated by Professor P. I. Branemark of Göteborg, Sweden.

In 1981 Dr. Fredrickson, along with Dr. Kenji Higuchi, oral and maxillofacial surgeon from Spokane, Washington, were invited to Göteborg, Sweden, as members of a surgical prosthetic team to receive training in the Branemark system. Three American teams participated in the revolutionary type of dental implant therapy, which included 5 days of intensive training in surgical, clinical prosthetic, and technical aspects of the Branemark system of osseointegration of dental implants.

Shortly after he returned to Spokane, Dr. Fredrickson, whose private practice principally was devoted to prosthodontics and maxillofacial prosthetics, applied his newly acquired knowledge of the Branemark system of osseointegrated dental implants to treat edentulous patients—thus becoming the first dentist in private practice in the United States to use this modality of dental implantation. Dr. Fredrickson and his clinical-technical team may be considered as apostles of osseointegration.

Dr. Fredrickson was a founder and charter member of the Academy of Maxillofacial Prosthetics and served as president. He also served as president of the American Prosthodontic Society. He and his team have contributed to many scientific programs with innovative and clinically relevant presentations. Dr. Fredrickson's primary motivation in writing (along with his fellow authors) the book on implant treatment is to help the clinician and the dental technician achieve optimal results, with a practical, sensible *hands-on* approach that is based on the actual treatment of patients.

The text is a teaching manual that is an essential, basic document for the student in the discipline of implant prosthodontics. It reflects the most current, accepted information on clinical and technical procedures in dental implant treatment.

The objective of the text is to educate the dentist, the dental staff, and the dental technician in the clinical and technical phases of implant treatment for the edentulous and the partially edentulous patient. With the passage of time, advances in dental implant treatment mandate documentation of new information. The application of new knowledge based on clinical experience must include laboratory and technical procedures to support and improve clinical procedures. The acquisition of clinical and technical prosthodontic knowledge applied to implant treatment is a critical factor in providing comfort, function, and health to the patient.

Edward J. Fredrickson's professional life has been devoted to helping his fellowman by his complete dedication to the treatment of patients. This remarkable, comprehensive text epitomizes the skill, knowledge, and experience of a master clinician in the organization of treatment procedures for dental implants. During my 40 years of close association with him, he has consistently exemplified the sterling qualities of a true professional. He has applied his skills with great competency. He lectures with clarity and a straightforward projection that confirms his knowledge and experience. He writes with skill about a complex and dramatic subject.

This book is a testament to excellence in practice by the documentation of clinical and technical procedures in the treatment of a broad spectrum of patients by implant therapy. Implant dentistry has developed considerably in the last decade. Materials, techniques, principles, and practices have evolved, significantly improving the quality and safety of implants, as an acceptable modality in dental health care.

I. Kenneth Adisman, D.D.S., M.S.

Preface

The importance of proper communication and coordination between the restorative dentist and the oral surgeon in both the surgical and prosthetic phases of the osseous implant-retained prosthesis is critical. To further state this importance, the success of the implant prosthesis must include the technical expertise and communication of the dental technician. This *team* concept has become my forte and is the underpinning of the significant rate of success with the implant prosthesis that has been delivered to the patients within the Spokane practice.

After I returned from Sweden, it became apparent that the success of the implant prosthesis should not rely only on the expertise of the restorative dentist but also should encompass a specialist in each field of the implant prosthesis's design and fabrication: the *team*.

The dental technician charged with the laboratory phases of the implant prosthesis must be well versed in all phases of fixed and removable prosthodontics. Mr. Maurice L. Gress, C.D.T., F.N.B.C., of AU Dental Ceramics in Spokane, accepted the challenge of the technical fabrication of the implant prosthesis. He trained and worked side-by-side with Dr. Tomas Jansson, Dr. Branemark's colleague, during the fabrication of the first Branemark osseous implant prosthesis in the United States. The early years of the implant prosthesis fabrication were the conventional (hybrid) treatment planning; however, in 1985, when Dr. Patrick Stevens joined the Spokane practice, his extensive training and expertise in maxillofacial prosthodontics opened the doors for extensive research, design, and documentation of the fixed implant-retained prosthesis.

The implant-retained prosthesis must be designed and fabricated with the patient's well-being and welfare in mind. Habituating to a new prosthesis is a *new way of life* for the edentulous patient, but it is also a major investment of time and money. The patient expects the best effort and results; therefore, the restorative dentist and the dental laboratory technician must be prepared to deliver the quality result that is anticipated and deserved.

This book presents the clinical and dental laboratory procedures for the fabrication of tissue implanted prostheses, using the applications of full edentulous fixed, partially edentulous, single tooth restorations, and overdentures. It also includes a chapter on the hygiene maintenance of the implant prosthesis. The details of the clinical and laboratory fabrication of the implant prosthesis have evolved over a 10-year period, after the Branemark implant system was first introduced in the United States. Through trial and error our team has distinctly improved the original clinical and laboratory procedures.

Edward J. Fredrickson, D.D.S.

Acknowledgment

Our appreciation to Sandra K. Gress for the dedication, support, and persistence in compiling the data of this manuscript to its completed form.

Edward J. Fredrickson, D.D.S.
Patrick J. Stevens, D.D.S.
Maurice L. Gress, C.D.T., F.N.B.C.

Contents

IMPLANT PROSTHODONTICS
CLINICAL AND LABORATORY PROCEDURES

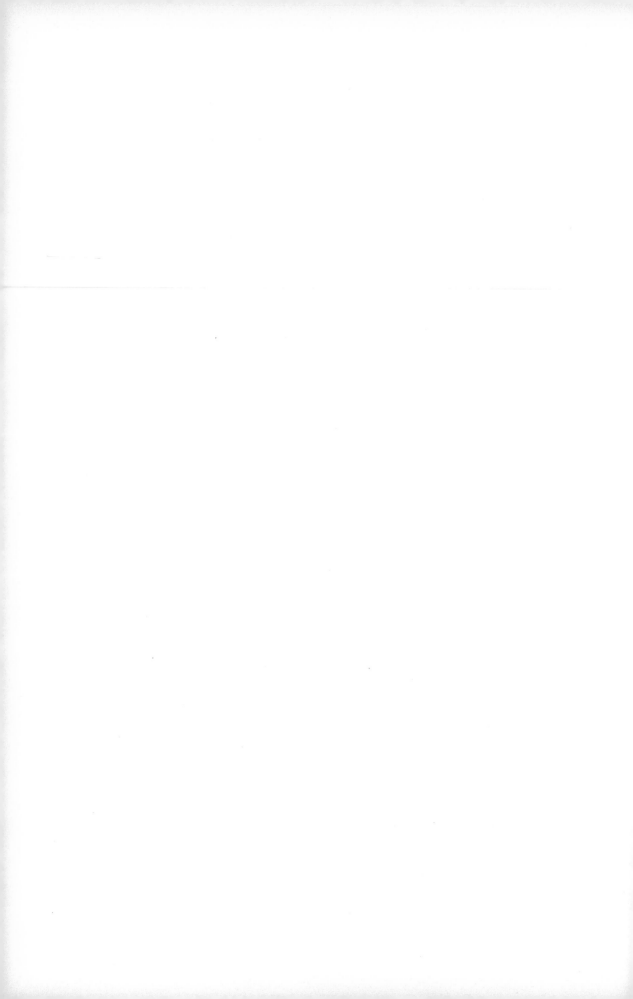

Loss of teeth, eventual edentulism, and the wearing of complete dentures have been part of the expected course of aging by the general population. The incidence of edentulism in the Western world has posed a challenge to prosthodontists and oral surgeons, encouraging them to devise acceptable prosthetic results for patients. Although the patient may adapt well to the complete denture prosthesis, the decrease in masticatory function, in comparison with that of complete natural dentition, has been well documented. Years of wearing complete dentures leads to progressive bone resorption. The resorptive process decreases surface area for prosthesis support, eliminates favorable anatomy for retention, and results in unfavorable denture-bearing areas. These results include unfavorably positioned muscle attachments, mental nerve sensitivity, and irregular bony configurations that underlie thin mucosa. Loss of lateral stability and retention increases prosthesis movement, resulting in increased friction and mucosal irritation.

Many surgical procedures have been developed over the years to restore more favorable anatomy for prosthesis support. Some of these include vestibuloplasty; vestibuloplasty, with skin or mucosal grafting; and augmentation, with either rib or hip bone grafting procedures. These procedures offered short-term improvement in denture stability and retention; however, none showed long-term clinical success.

Well-meaning-but-not-researched methods of implanting artificial material to aid in denture retention have been used for many years, with varying degrees of clinical success.

The first scientifically based study on the biocompatability of implantable materials began in Sweden in 1952. Animal studies, including work with rabbits and dogs, indicated that properly prepared surgical grade titanium in combination with careful surgical technique resulted in a predictable biologic response and a phenomenon that was termed *osseointegration* by its progenitor, Professor Per-Ingvar Branemark, Göteberg, Sweden.

Branemark defines the osseointegration process in his book, *Tissue Integrated Prostheses* as the "direct structural and functional connection between ordered, living bone and the surface of a load-carrying implant. Creation and maintenance of osseointegration, therefore, depends on the understanding of the tissue's healing, repair, and remodeling capacities." The first edentulous patients were treated in Sweden with titanium implants in 1965. The long-term clinical success of the Swedes and other international teams, who were following proper protocol, is well documented.[6]

The purpose of this book is to present clinical and laboratory techniques in the prosthetic rehabilitation of edentulous and partially edentulous patients. It entails 9 years of pictoral documentation of the clinical and laboratory procedures for implant prosthesis recipients, primarily within the private practices of Dr. Edward J. Fredrickson, Dr. Patrick J. Stevens, and Dr. Kenji Higuchi, with prosthesis fabrication by Fellow certified dental technician, Mr. Maurice L. Gress.

The team concept has allowed for the perfecting of clinical, chairside techniques and laboratory procedures. The fabrication of the implant prosthesis is not a simple task, and it should not be presumed that the procedure can be done quickly. In most cases the prosthesis is fabricated by a technician who is well versed in all phases of crown and bridge and ceramics and who is familiar with dentures.

Through the years the clinical and laboratory procedures that were used during this documentation were perfected as new materials were introduced to the industry; materials change, but no method exists that can expedite the fabrication procedures. The technician, as well as the doctor, must keep the well-being of the patient in mind. When the clinical staff is trained to understand the fabricating procedures, the patient, who is anxiously awaiting delivery of the prosthesis, can be reassured. The prosthesis introduces a new way of life for the edentulous patient; however, implant prosthodontics is a major investment.

The interdependence and communication between the restorative dentist and the dental laboratory technician are imperative to a successful prosthetic result and will be emphasized in the text. For this reason, this book is directed to the restorative dentist, undergraduate dental student, dental hygienist, dental technician, and dental assistant as a step-by-step handbook used for reference, not only in the classroom, but also in the clinic and laboratory.

1

Surgical Considerations in Implant Prosthodontics

Successful surgical-prosthetic treatment, using tissue integrated prostheses, requires an understanding of the biology of osseointegration. Branemark[6] introduced the concept of osseointegration, defining it as a direct structural and functional connection between ordered living bone and the surface of the load-carrying implant. Albrektsson[2] and others have outlined factors that can influence the creation and subsequent maintenance of an osseointegrated implant. This text focuses primarily on the prosthetic aspects of osseointegrated implant reconstruction; however, the dentist who performs the restorative surgery must comprehend the goals and limitations of surgery. The degree of surgical trauma, resulting from preparation of an implant recipient site, will greatly influence the capacity of osseous and soft tissues to remain differentiated and ultimately to support a prosthesis. Many authors[3,6,8,13] have addressed the scientific basis for osseointegration, which involves tissue healing and repair, component installation, and the remodeling response of the supporting bone to long-term functional demands. The two-stage surgical procedure that was introduced by Branemark has been reviewed by numerous authors.[1,6,12] A graphic description of the sequencing in fixture installation and abutment connection procedures is summarized in Fig. 1-1. A nondisturbed healing interval of 4 to 6 months takes place between the two procedures and depends primarily on whether surgery is performed in the mandible or in the maxilla.[6] This section will concentrate on the clinical aspects of surgery only as they relate to the prosthetic phase of treatment. For specific surgical technique the reader is referred to other sources. To improve clarity the author has chosen to limit the use of the generic word *implant* and instead will refer to the specific terms, *fixture* and *abutment,* to identify the bone anchoring component and the separately attached mucosa penetrating connector (Fig. 1-2). Although the content of this chapter is based upon the Branemark method of osseointegration, many of the principles expressed may also apply to alternatively designed implant systems.

Patient Assessment

The use of bone-anchored implants to secure an oral prosthesis should be provided only after thorough patient evaluation and planning. Few systemic health conditions prohibit the use of tissue integrated reconstruction. The patient must be able to tolerate the use of local anesthesia and intravenous sedation. Preexisting systemic diseases or prescribed medications that may interfere with this approach should

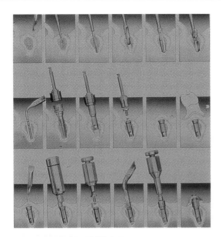

Fig. 1-1

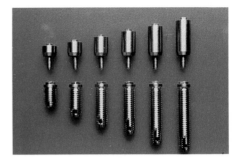

Fig. 1-2

be adequately reviewed and managed preoperatively. The absence of surface and subsurface pathology involving the soft and osseous tissues must be verified before surgery. Regional and local anatomic features need to be studied to determine the feasibility of implant placement. The patient's motivation for treatment, as well as a stable patient psyche, are critical psychologic aspects of patient selection. Unrealistic expectations of treatment or psychotic syndromes contraindicate treatment, regardless of favorable clinical indications.

In most situations, patient assessment and treatment planning involve a team approach, including a surgeon, a restorative dentist, and a dental technician. In specific instances, specialist consultation and treatment may involve the participation of the oral and maxillofacial surgeon, the prosthodontist, the periodontist, the orthodontist, as well as the restorative dentist. It is imperative to work with a trained dental laboratory technician, who is committed to performing his or her work precisely and who is familiar with the biomechanics of bone-anchored prosthesis design. Close collaboration among these individuals is essential when selecting patients and treatment plans, as well as during the actual clinical and technical procedures.

Clinical Examination

Despite scientific advances in various computer-imaging technology, a thorough clinical examination is foremost in determining the feasibility of fixture placement. In addition to a complete routine oral examination, specific attention should be directed to the following areas:

1. Inspection of the soft tissues overlying areas of potential fixture placement
2. Ridge or occlusal relationship to opposing arch
3. Vertical dimension and intermaxillary space
4. Arch length available for fixture placement
5. Alveolar ridge contour and width, as determined by bimanual palpation

Surface pathology, such as *epuli fissurata,* inflammatory hyperplasia, and white lesions over potential recipient sites, should be managed appropriately before fixture placement. Although it is not routinely necessary, it may be beneficial to consider a limited vestibuloplasty, using a palatal mucosal graft to minimize alveolar mucosal movement caused by unfavorable muscle activity.

A major responsibility of the operating surgeon relates to proper fixture placement. The osseointegration method is based upon careful and gentle handling of tissues, with minimal tissue damage, in a clean and aseptic operating environment. Although the creation of long-term, fixture-to-bone anchorage remains paramount, it is important to recognize that incorrectly placed fixtures, even if osseointegrated, may not be usable and thereby may result in failure.[20] Malpositioned fixtures can interfere with desirable prosthesis and framework design, access for oral hygiene, speech production, and optimal esthetics in the final prosthesis. The restorative dentist will design the final appearance of the prosthesis; however, it is the surgeon's responsibility to anticipate potential problems and limitations that may interfere with acceptable esthetic results. The anterior maxilla is the most critical area; regional soft tissue and bony morphology may affect the emergence profile and appearance of the final prosthesis. Parel and Sullivan[16] have emphasized that careful attention must be paid to maxillary labial plate contour. Loss of the labial plate, as a result of trauma or tooth removal, can affect optimal fixture positioning, as well as cause contour and symmetry problems of the emerging restoration. Residual ridge contour defects involving the soft tissues and residual bony alveolus may be improved, using a variety of augmentation procedures, with mucosa, bone, or alloplastic materials. Assessment of the patient's upper lip position with the mouth in repose, during smiling, and during facial expression activity is important when determining the expectations and limitations of the cosmetic results.

Proper conventional fixture placement requires attention, both to spacing (mesial-distal) and to angulation (buccal-lingual). When possible, it is ideal to position fixtures in sites where teeth are planned in the final, implant-retained, fixed prosthesis (Fig. 1-3). Fixtures placed interproximally, or in the embrasure areas of the final prosthesis, usually will compromise esthetics and present oral maintenance problems for the patient. Fixture and abutment units that are spaced too closely have occasionally led to interabutment tissue hyperplasia. Fixtures overangulated toward the labial can cause a disharmonious emergence profile from the alveolar ridge when they are compared to adjacent teeth and can necessitate the screw access opening to be placed on the labial surface of the final restoration. Excessive palatal or lingual angulation of fixtures may require that the prosthestic framework be bulky, interfering with speech function and cleaning access. Precise fixture placement depends on the patient's existing anatomy, the skill and experience of the operating surgeon, and an adequate preoperative plan, using the team concept.

The ridge relationship to the opposing arch, either dentate or edentulous, influences buccal-lingual positioning (angulation) of the fixture(s), with respect to the desired final prosthesis. Physical examination, cephalometric findings, and evaluation of mounted diagnostic casts provide information regarding ridge and jaw relationship. If a skeletal maxillo-mandibular disharmony exists, then orthognathic surgery should be considered before, or at the same time as, fixture placement. Excessive fixture angulation to accommodate severe Class II or Class III ridge relationships may result in anterior fixtures directed into lip anatomy or into the floor of the mouth (Fig. 1-4). The opposing occlusion, either artificial or natural, can be an effective guide for fixture positioning, particularly in the edentulous situation (Fig. 1-5).

For the patient who is partially edentulate, a limited intermaxillary space in centric occlusion may prohibit or compromise implant reconstruction (Fig. 1-6). Ideally, intermaxillary space not only should adequately accommodate the abutment unit and prosthetic framework, but also should permit correct anatomic tooth replacement. If the opposing dentition has supererupted into an edentulous area, it may be necessary to establish again the proper occlusal plane prosthetically or to perform orthodontic treatment to idealize the interarch space. Frequently, in areas of potential fixture-abutment sites, the residual alveolar process is noted to have adequate vertical height but is unfavorably thin in a buccal-palatal or buccal-lingual dimension. The Branemark-designed fixture has a diameter of 3.75 mm and would theoretically require a bone width of at least 4.00 mm to accommodate the fixture. With adequate experience the clinician, using bimanual palpation, can develop tactile and proprioceptive skills to subjectively assess the feasibility of fixture installation relative to ridge width in the maxilla and posterior mandible. Direct measurement of alveolar width can be made using mucosal penetrating calipers with local anesthesia (Fig. 1-7). The available mesial-distal arch length in the partially edentulous jaw can be measured either directly or on the diagnostic study casts. The design of the final prosthesis, the available mesial-distal arch length, and the residual bony anatomy are all factors in planning the number of fixtures that will be used. Computed tomography is helpful in defining morphologic features and bone volume.

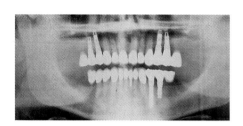

Fig. 1-3

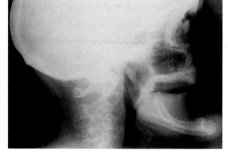

Fig. 1-4

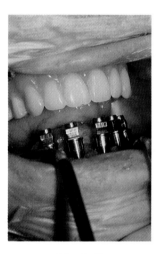

Fig. 1-5

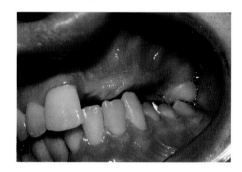

Fig. 1-6

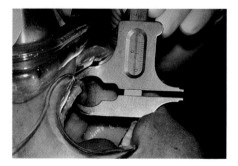

Fig. 1-7

As a consesquence of long-term edentulism, hypodontia, cleft conditions, congential aplasia, traumatic injuries, or oncologic defects, complex jawbone anatomy may not permit conventional fixture placement. When the residual bone volume (width and height) is deficient, bone graft augmentation may be appropriate. A number of surgical approaches for bone graft augmentation have been advocated using onlay, nasal floor, and sinus grafting.[10,14,19] Many of these procedures are in the beginnings of their development and are recommended only for specific defect anatomy. Currently, additional research in the area of tissue-guided regeneration, using synthetic membranes, is in progress.[7,15] This concept, as well as the use of osteoinductive materials, may help in the future management of less-than-optimal bony anatomy and may extend the limits of treatment.

Radiologic Examination

Initial radiographic examination will vary if the patient is edentulate or partially dentate. An orthopantomogram and a lateral cephalometric film will usually provide adequate imaging for most of the patients who are endentulate. Information regarding local bony pathology, general bone volume and quality, and anteroposterior jaw relationship can be obtained. In the patient who is partially edentulate, an orthopantomogram—a full-mouth periapical series—and, if indicated, occlusal films are screening studies. Morphologic jaw shape and bone quality are assessed. Lekholm and Zarb[6] have characterized radiographic appearance in terms of bone quality. Dense trabecular bone in combination with varying thicknesses of compact bone is suggestive of good bone quality, while a thin layer of cortical bone over low-density trabecular bone implies poor bone quality. Frost[9] has demonstrated that each skeletal tissue type displays different mechanical strength characteristics, based on mechanical unit load values. Bone quality is a factor in achieving primary fixture stability at the time of placement, and prosthetically, bone of limited quality should not be subjected to excessive occlusal load demands before remodeling is completed (at least 18 months). In circumstances involving extreme defect anatomy, when precise dimensional configuration is needed, or before mandibular fixture surgery that requires localization of the inferior alveolar nerve, computed tomography is often indicated. Schwartz[11,17,18] and others have advocated the use of reformatted multiplanar computed tomography in obtaining cross-sectional imaging to accurately define the shape, height, and width of the maxilla and mandible at potential fixture sites (Figs. 1-8 and 1-9). This information is of value in developing a surgical treatment plan and the feasibility of fixture positioning.

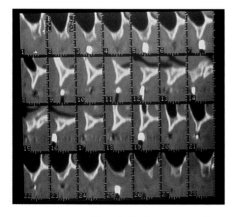

Fig. 1-8, A

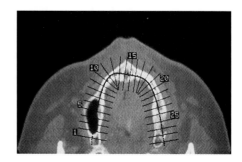

Fig. 1-8, B

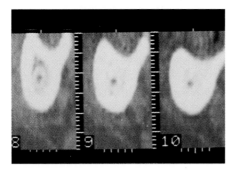

Fig. 1-9, A

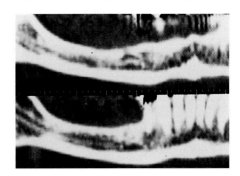

Fig. 1-9, B

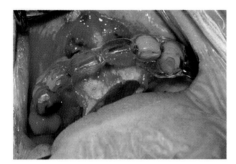

Fig. 1-10, A

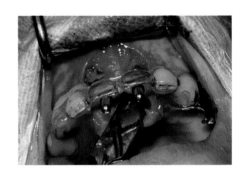

Fig. 1-10, B

Treatment Planning

Close communication between the operating surgeon, the restorative dentist, and the dental technician is essential to develop a coordinated treatment plan following consultation, physical evaluation, and review of appropriate imaging studies. The patient's concerns and desires should be reviewed before providing an implant-supported prosthesis. Diagnostic study casts mounted on a semiadjustable articulator will assist in planning and designing the final prosthesis. The number and location of potential fixtures should be identified, and the anticipated abutment type should be decided. The potential surgical, prosthetic, and technical difficulties should be discussed. Temporary or relined prostheses must be accurate, relative to anterior tooth position, to fully guide the surgeon in fixture installation. A well-designed, temporary prosthesis, or a waxing of the planned final prosthesis can be used to fabricate a surgical template. Several designs of surgical templates (stents) are possible and are intended to direct the surgeon in optimal fixture spacing and angulation based on final prosthesis design. Fig. 1-10, *A*, is an example of an easily fabricated vacuum-formed, surgical template that defines labial contours of the proposed final prosthesis. This can serve to assist both in mesial-distal site placement, as well as the buccal-lingual or buccal-palatal angulation of the fixture (Fig. 1-10, *B*).

The final surgical-prosthetic treatment plan must consider the training, experience, and skills of the surgeon, the restorative dentist, and the dental technician. In acquiring new technical skills, all clinicians follow an individual learning curve that influences their performance of the skill. Experience, training, and aptitude are factors in the progress along this learning curve. Henry[3] has made some general recommendations in the surgical management of dental applications of osseointegration with reference to specialty and nonspecialty dentists. Those who have limited experience and training should seek out assistance and initially restrict their activities to routine and straightforward cases. More demanding clinical situations should be referred or delayed until adequate expertise is acquired. *Patients with complex defect anatomy are best treated by using a specialist team approach. It is clear that the principle of placing the patient's best interest first should be foremost.*

The placement of a tissue implant–retained prosthesis can potentially result in a lifelong reconstruction and can provide significant functional and psychologic benefits for the patient. Surgical, restorative, and laboratory team members must accept the serious responsibility that entails properly plannning and placing fixtures, fabricating the prosthesis, and maintaining the osseointegrated reconstruction so that such lofty goals are possible.

2

Diagnostic/Surgical Stents

Team Communication and Treatment Planning

Even at an early age, many have experienced being a member of a *team,* whether it was a sports oriented team or a scholastically originated one. As an individual's career path evolves, often there are those who are instrumental in helping that person achieve his or her goals. As much as many like to think of themselves as self-reliant individualists, most are members of some type of team.

In the medical and dental professions the team concept has always been present, but since the fixed implant retained prosthesis has become a method of choice for edentulous restoration, the *team* has expanded and now incorporates the restorative dentist, the oral surgeon, and the dental laboratory technician. Team communication and preparation among the restorative dentist, the oral surgeon, and the dental laboratory technician are essential for the best possible results in implant prosthetics. Treatment planning will eliminate costly errors for all concerned. Fig.s 2-1 through 2-6 are examples of poor treatment planning. Note that the arch form has been neglected by placement of fixtures in a straight line, that there is radical and diverging angulation, that the screw access channels are exiting through facial surfaces, that the fixtures are placed too close together for proper prosthesis design and hygiene, and that there are too few fixtures to balance both quadrants of the arch. All of these problem areas could have been eliminated through proper treatment planning and evaluation by the doctors and the dental technician.

Treatment Planning

Fixture placement is crucial. Part of the close teamwork between the oral surgeon, the restorative dentist, and the dental technician is to ensure that the position of fixture placement is correct. Treatment planning will idealize patient treatment physiologically and psychologically. As mentioned in Chapter 1, physiological considerations include an assessment of the overall health of the patient, the local health condition of the patient's jaws and mucosa membranes, and the morphological features of the operative area. Pathological conditions must not be present around the bone tissue. Other physiological considerations include whether active or hyperactive gag reflexes are elicited by a removable prosthesis, even when adequate denture retention or stability is present. The patient should be informed whether the implant prosthesis can be designed to look like natural dentition or like the compromise of it. Sometimes this compromise is necessary because of excessive bone resorption. If the patient is aware of all the circumstances surrounding the design of the prosthesis, the expectation level will be pleasingly satisfactory for all involved.

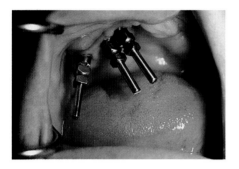

Fig. 2-1

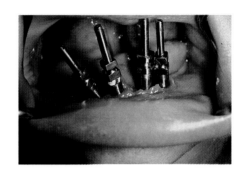

Fig. 2-2

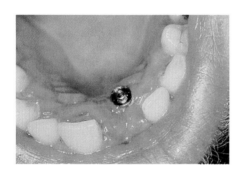

Fig. 2-3

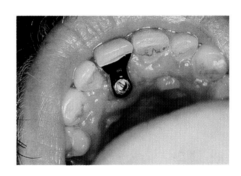

Fig. 2-4

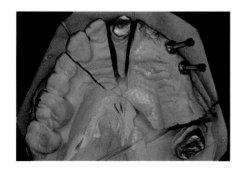

Fig. 2-5

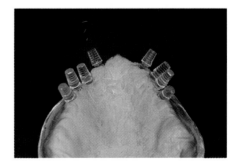

Fig. 2-6

Diagnostic Stent

A diagnostic stent is fabricated to facilitate ideal fixture placement for the restorative dentist and the oral surgeon. The diagnostic stent may be used in conjunction with the radiograph to evaluate the vertical bone height and the location of the mental foramen in the mandible where the nerve canal lies. In the maxilla, the diagnostic stent evaluates bone height and floor of the nose. It does not project shape, density, or quality of the bone. This projection can only be determined through radiographical and surgical evaluation. A number of configurations can be used, depending on application of the desired prosthesis. A simple method for placing the full maxilla or mandible diagnostic stent is achieved by securing, with sticky wax, a 4 mm ball bearing on the external surface of the stent in close proximity to where the fixtures will be implanted (Fig. 2-7). For single tooth or partially edentulous cases where a removable prosthesis is not present, a custom diagnostic stent is fabricated by impressing the tissue (Fig. 2-8), mounting the cast (Fig. 2-9), using acrylic denture teeth for a partial setup (Fig. 2-10), carrying the baseplate wax over the occlusal and incisal edges and over the existing teeth, and processing in clear acrylic (Fig. 2-11). On reclaiming and finishing, 4 mm steel ball bearings are placed in the stent at desired fixture sites (Fig. 2-12). The stent is placed in the oral cavity. Radiographs are used to aid in fixture placement (Figs. 2-13 and 2-14).

Analyzation of the radiograph by the restorative dentist, the oral surgeon, and the dental technician will determine the prosthesis options that will be discussed with the patient. It is important that these options, as well as the esthetic and functional expectations, are understood by the patient. Total patient awareness of the pros and cons of the procedure will eliminate misunderstanding and frustration when the prosthesis is delivered.

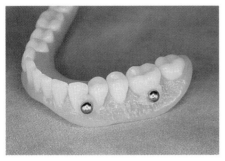

Fig. 2-7

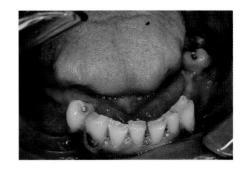

Fig. 2-8

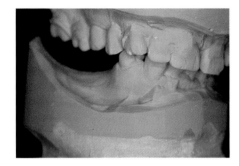

Fig. 2-9

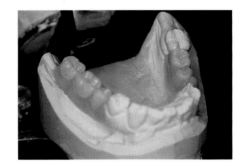

Fig. 2-10

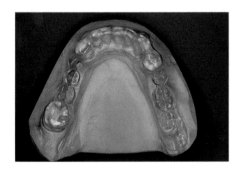

Fig. 2-11

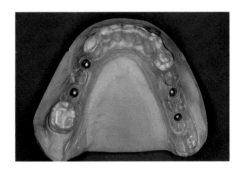

Fig. 2-12

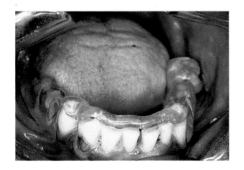

Fig. 2-13

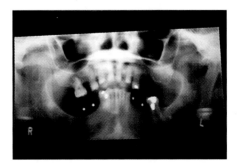

Fig. 2-14

Surgical Stent

After the treatment plan has been determined by both the restorative dentist and oral surgeon, a surgical stent is fabricated by the dental technician. The desired configuration of the surgical stent is determined by the prescribed prosthesis. In most applications the diagnostic stent may be altered for use in the implant surgery (Fig. 2-15). This alteration is accomplished by relieving the inferior border of the appliance 3 mm to 4 mm to allow the surgeon room for soft tissue reflection. Other fabrication methods include making an impression of the tissue, taking interocclusal records, and pouring a master cast plaster. An impression is also made of the opposing arch. If the opposing arch is edentulous, an impression and cast are made of the denture for a trial denture setup. The casts are mounted on an adjustable articulator, using a centric relation record at an acceptable occlusal vertical dimension (Fig. 2-16). The most posterior sites for the fixture placement are set in relation to the mandibular mental foramen bilaterally (Fig. 2-17). These sites are identified and reference marks are made on the cast. The anterior residual ridge between the reference points is blocked out between the labial and the lingual sulci, using three layers of baseplate wax (Fig. 2-18). This relief area will allow the surgical stent to be completely seated on the posterior ridge and will not interfere with the sutured tissue in the anterior area. For ease of separation an impression of the relief cast is taken and then duplicated in laboratory plaster (Fig. 2-19). A vacuum-forming machine is used to adapt a single layer of 0.080 inch plastic sheet material over this duplicate cast (Fig. 2-20). The excess material is trimmed and the borders are adjusted to the cast and finished in a similar procedure as a denture border. Guide pin holes are drilled through the relief area for the fixture placement by the oral surgeon (Fig. 2-21). The stent is then verified on the mounted diagnostic cast before delivery to the oral surgeon (Fig. 2-22). Another method for producing a stent is to take an impression of the existing prosthesis and duplicate it in acrylic (Fig. 2-23). Guide pin holes are placed for the position and angulation of fixtures (Fig. 2-24). Fig. 2-25 shows the duplication of the maxilla obtaining a bite relationship to the edentulous mandible. Steel guides are placed to indicate fixture position and angulation (Fig. 2-26). This method is unique because it does not interfere with the reflection of tissue during surgery. There are additional applications of the surgical stent for the single tooth prosthesis (Figs. 2-27 through 2-30), the anterior partially edentulous prosthesis (Figs. 2-31 through 2-34), and the posterior unilateral and bilateral partially edentulous prosthesis.

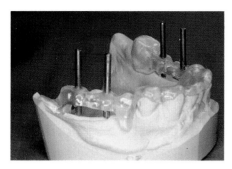

Fig. 2-15

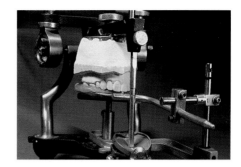

Fig. 2-16

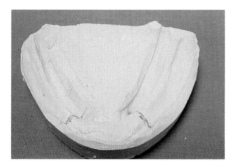

Fig. 2-17

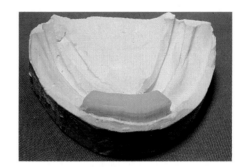

Fig. 2-18

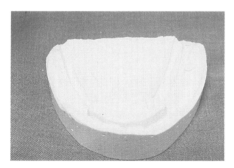

Fig. 2-19

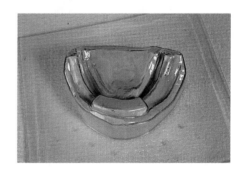

Fig. 2-20

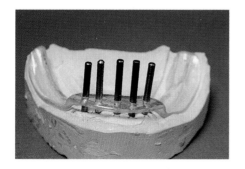

Fig. 2-21

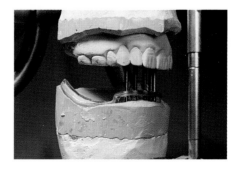

Fig. 2-22

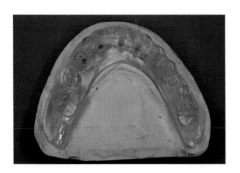

Fig. 2-23

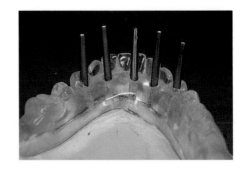

Fig. 2-24

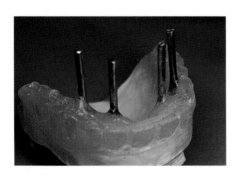

Fig. 2-25

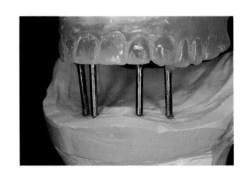

Fig. 2-26

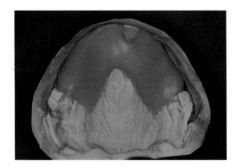

Fig. 2-27

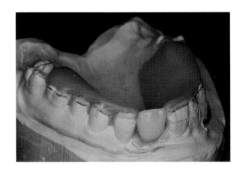

Fig. 2-28

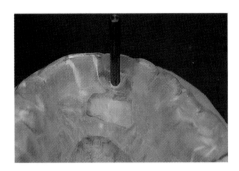

Fig. 2-29

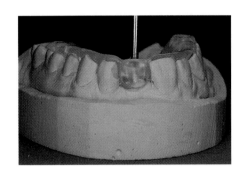

Fig. 2-30

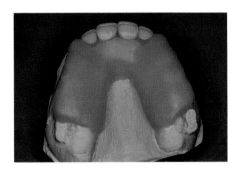

Fig. 2-31

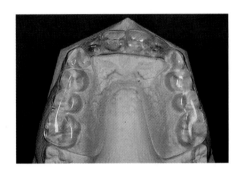

Fig. 2-32

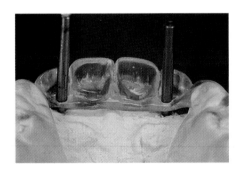

Fig. 2-33

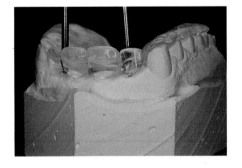

Fig. 2-34

3

Completely Edentulous Fixed Implant-Retained Prosthesis—Mandibular Arch

Most complaints about dentures come from patients who are completely edentulous on the mandibular arch. Resorption of the alveolar ridge results in decreased surface area and anatomical configuration, which lessens denture retention and stability. The increase in movement of the lower denture results in mucosal irritation and ulceration, reducing masticatory efficiency and increasing patient discomfort. As the mandibular resorptive process continues, the denture may impinge on the mental foramen and nerve and on the genial tubercles, which may hamper prosthesis use altogether.

When a patient first complains about the mandibular denture, a thorough evaluation of the existing prosthesis is made. This procedure includes an evaluation of the proper denture extensions, the dental occlusion, and the vertical dimension of the occlusion. The patient is given a head and neck evaluation, including a cancer screening, as well as a radiographic and an intraoral examination are completed and charted. Health history questionnaires are administered and followed by an in-depth patient interview. The patient's previous denture history is charted to evaluate his or her expectations. The process of patient awareness and prosthesis education is given, informing the patient of the many prosthetic options. The patient's choices include having no treatment, relining an existing prosthesis, making a new prosthesis, or fabricating one of the various implant-supported prostheses. Different prosthetic options shown in literature, in dental models, or in videotapes are helpful for patient education. If the patient is interested in pursuing a tissue-integrated prosthesis, a referral is made for surgical evaluation.

After the surgeon has evaluated the amount of bone the patient has available and the number of implants that can be predictably placed, a second consultation is scheduled to determine the best prosthetic option for the patient from a functional, esthetic, hygienic, and financial standpoint. The patient's dexterity, finger strength, and motivation for hygiene may influence the prosthetic option. If the patient's dexterity for hygiene and his or her finances are not a consideration, the fixed mandibular implant prosthesis may be the treatment of choice.

With a prosthesis of any kind, advantages and disadvantages exist. The advantages of the tissue-integrated fixed prosthesis compared with an implant-retained overdenture are:

1. Lack of tissue contact

No mucosal support is required with the fixed-implant prosthesis. The fixture abutment unit supports the prosthesis completely, allowing no tooth movement. This eliminates any potential tissue irritation from prosthesis movement.

2. Increased masticatory efficiency

The implant-retained fixed prosthesis is established similarly to that of natural dentition. The only limitation to chewing is from the maxilla, if removable prosthetics are present.

3. Psychological advantage

Tooth loss and the wearing of a complete denture are often associated with aging. Some patients have moderate-to-severe psychological problems regarding edentulism or using a removable prosthesis. The fixed prosthesis eliminates a removable prosthesis and greatly enhances the patient's self-image and self-confidence.

Disadvantages of the fixed implant prosthesis include:

1. Lack of tissue support

Many patients who have complete dentures have undergone considerable resorption of the mandible. The denture was used to reestablish lip support and contours. The mental labial fold has often been eliminated by the removable prosthesis, and the patient has become accustomed to this appearance. The length of the cantilever distance is measured from the distal surface of the distal-most fixture on each side. The maximum cantilever recommended is 15 mm. This distance may leave the patient in first molar occlusion and with a lack of tooth support in the mandibular posterior.

2. Complication from component breakage and fixture loss

Component breakage and complications are more common with the fixed prosthesis caused in part by the forces generated in the cantilevered section of the prosthesis. Fixture loss may require shortening the implant prosthesis or converting to an overdenture prosthesis.

3. Complicated procedures

The clinical and laboratory procedures are technically more demanding with the tissue-integrated prosthesis in comparison with the overdenture prosthesis.

4. Expense

The patient cost for surgical and prosthetic procedures of the implant prosthesis may be several thousand dollars more than for an overdenture or removable prosthesis because of the following reasons: (a) more fixtures and components are used; (b) the number and length of clinical appointments for prosthetic completion are increased; and (c) the technical procedures of the laboratory are more specialized and a higher degree of expertise is required.

5. Hygiene

The contours of the implant prosthesis may prove difficult for patients with poor eyesight, limited dexterity, or lack of motivation to maintain a plaque-free tooth environment.

Clinical and Laboratory Procedures

Clinical

Procedures for the mandibular fixed-implant retained prosthesis begin 7 to 10 days after the fixture placements. The patient has a transitional denture fabricated to establish phonetics and esthetics at the proper vertical dimension of occlusion. The transitional denture is used to evaluate the patient's temporomandibular joint response to the vertical dimension of occlusion and as a guide for fabrication of the surgical stent. After suture removal and adequate tissue healing have occurred, a tissue conditioner is used to reline the mandibular denture. The denture is relieved in the area corresponding to the flap reflection. The tissue conditioning material is mixed and applied, the denture seated, border molded, and the patient is guided into centric relation occlusion. After the recommended set time, the denture is removed and placed in a pressure pot at 20 pounds per square inch (psi) in warm water for 10 minutes. The excess material is trimmed and the denture polished. The denture is worn and tissue treatment material is replaced as needed until complete healing has occurred. A processed methylmethacrylate resin reline is completed, and the denture is worn until the second phase surgery is performed. The patient is advised to seek denture adjustment for all tissue irritation to prevent fixture exposure. For the mandible, 4 months is the average healing period before the abutment surgery is completed.

Seven to 10 days after the second phase surgery the transitional mandibular denture is again tissue treated as previously described, except that now the denture is relieved adequately to allow clearance around the transmucosal abutments and healing caps. Preliminary impressions of the maxilla and mandible are made, using an alginate impression material in stock edentulous impression trays (Figs. 3-1 and 3-2).

The preliminary alginate impression is cast in dental stone and trimmed for the preparation of the custom tray fabrication (Fig. 3-3).

Custom Tray Fabrication

The custom tray is used to make an impression that will provide an accurate recording of the mandibular or maxillary tissues and their relationship to the integrated fixtures.

This tray is different from a standard edentulous tray in that it has openings that are designed to allow access to the guide pins and impression copings. The impression copings and guide pins are picked up in the impression material that is confined within the tray. This impression provides an accurate relation of the fixtures to one another and to the surrounding oral tissues.

Baseplate wax is used to provide relief in the buccal, lingual, and distal areas to the abutments on the cast for custom tray fabrication (Fig. 3-4). A single layer of baseplate wax is used as a relief in the distal extension areas. Sufficient wax relief is achieved by a strip of baseplate wax 8 mm wide × 6 mm high (Fig. 3-5) over the crest of the residual ridge and over the abutment fixture area. The ridge is then smoothed with a wax spatula.

The custom tray material is molded over the cast, and the fixture area is reinforced with excess resin (Figs. 3-6 and 3-7). A laboratory knife is used to cut a window over the occlusal portion of the abutment relief area and allowed to completely polymerize (Fig. 3-8).

After polymerization the custom tray is removed from the preliminary cast and borders are trimmed for a conventional denture (Fig. 3-9). The tray is placed on the cast and verified for a minimum clearance of 3 mm between the custom tray and the replica area of the abutment. If the clearance is acceptable, it is finished, polished, and sent to the clinic for final impressions (Fig. 3-10).

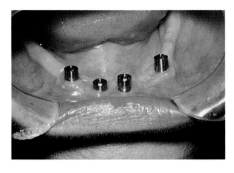

Fig. 3-1

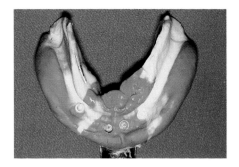

Fig. 3-2

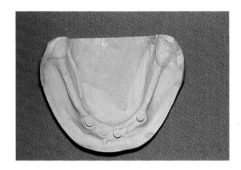

Fig. 3-3

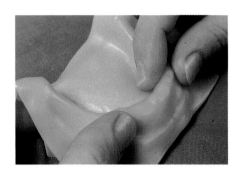

Fig. 3-4

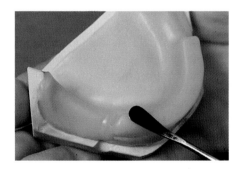

Fig. 3-5

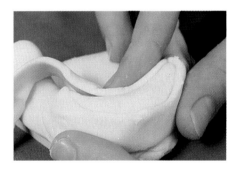

Fig. 3-6

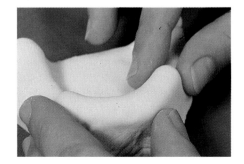

Fig. 3-7

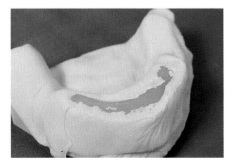

Fig. 3-8

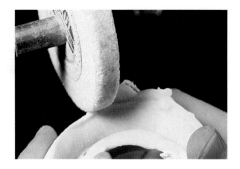

Fig. 3-9

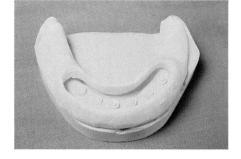

Fig. 3-10

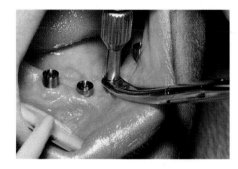

Fig. 3-11

Clinical Final Impression Procedures

Titanium hemostats and the hexagonal wrench are used to ensure abutment screw tightness (Fig. 3-11). Impression copings are attached to the abutments with the proper length guide pins (Fig. 3-12). The square impression copings are preferred because they resist rotation and displacement in the impression material. The open window custom tray is tried in the mouth for comfort and path of insertion (Fig. 3-13). The abutment, impression coping, and guide pin angulation and/or interference may necessitate adjustment of the tray dimension to allow insertion. Baseplate wax is sealed over the window, and the tray is heated in a water bath, and then inserted over the guide pins and impression copings (Fig. 3-14).

The guide pins should penetrate the wax to allow access for removal of the impression (Figs. 3-15 and 3-16). The tray is painted with the appropriate adhesive, and the impression material of choice is mixed to manufacturer's specifications. The impression material should be a medium viscosity mix that will flow through a syringe and should have a stiff set (Fig. 3-17). A vinyl polysiloxane impression material is recommended. After the impression is mixed, the material is loaded into the tray and the syringe. The material is first injected around the impression copings, and the tray is seated, using the guide pins and holes in the wax window as a guide for placement. Ideally, the guide pins should all penetrate the wax window, and the screw slots in the guide pins should be accessible. Excess impression material is cleared from the guide pins before complete setting. After the impression material has set, the guide pins are accessed and then unscrewed with a screwdriver of the appropriate length (Figs. 3-18 and 3-19). The guide pins are unscrewed until two or three clicks are heard, which indicate a complete guide pin disconnection. The guide pins are left in the same holes in the impression to allow accurate placement of the abutment replicas. Final impressions of the maxilla are completed at this time, also.

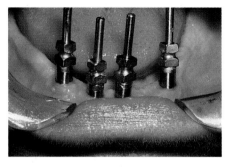

Fig. 3-12

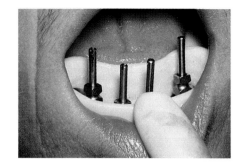

Fig. 3-13

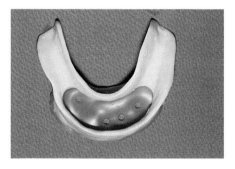

Fig. 3-14

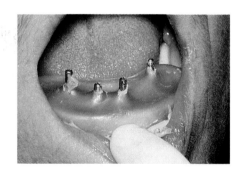

Fig. 3-15

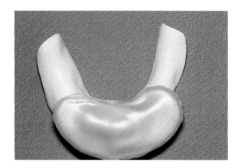

Fig. 3-16

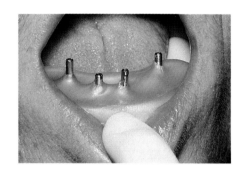

Fig. 3-17

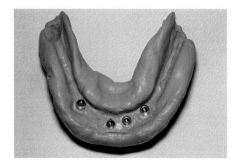

Fig. 3-18

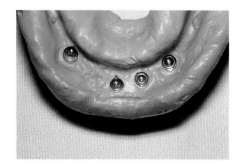

Fig. 3-19

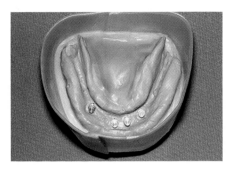

Fig. 3-20

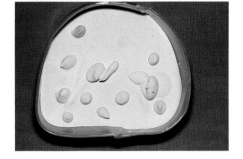

Fig. 3-21

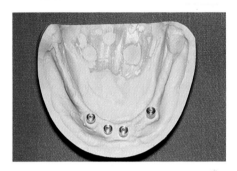

Fig. 3-22

Master Cast, Verification Stent, and Wax Rim

The master cast is the foundation for fabricating the implant prosthesis. Therefore, the dental technician must use methodical procedures that will ensure an accurate reproduction of the intraoral tissues.

Brass replicas have been precisely machined to be analogues of the superior surface of the abutment. The replicas are screwed onto the impression copings with guide pins. *Extreme* caution must be used not to entrap any foreign material between the brass replica and the impression coping interface. Foreign material may cause inaccuracy in the master cast, which will subsequently be transferred to the framework.

After the placement of the brass replicas, the final impression is beaded with utility wax and boxed with wax strips in the usual manner (Fig. 3-20). The impression is cast in vacuum-mixed diestone. Retention for the second pour is placed in the distal extension areas (Fig. 3-21). The anterior region around the replicas is left flat for cast alterations (if necessary) after framework trial fitting. When the first pour has set, a base in yellow stone is poured (Fig. 3-22). Each guide pin must be completely unscrewed until the characteristic click is heard two or three times before separating the impression from the cast. Elimination of this step may cause fracturing to the cast or damage to the impression.

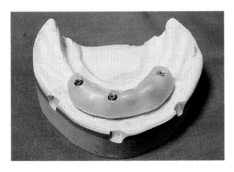

Fig. 3-23

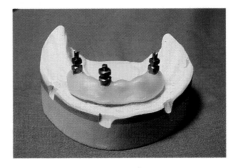

Fig. 3-24

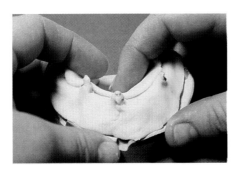

Fig. 3-25

Occlusion Rim Fabrication

Maxillomandibular relations are recorded, using a customized record base and an interocclusal rim. The record base is stabilized by incorporating gold cylinders or impression copings into the record base. This base is unique because it can be secured in the mouth with guide pins for recording centric relation and vertical dimension of occlusion.

The occlusion rim is fabricated on the master cast. Gold cylinders or impression copings are placed on two or three of the abutment replicas on the master cast. Placement on the anterior abutments facilitates access during clinical trial fittings.

One thickness of baseplate wax is adapted around the replicas and extended slightly beyond the most distal replicas. Three replicas are located and exposed through the block-out wax, and guide pins are screwed into the impression copings (Figs. 3-23 and 3-24).

Undesirable undercuts on the master cast are blocked out with baseplate wax. A tin foil substitute is placed on the exposed areas of the stone and an autopolymerizing resin is mixed according to manufacturer's directions, rolled out, and adapted to the master cast (Fig. 3-25). The tray material must engage undercuts in the gold cylinders or impression copings. A double thickness of resin is added to the lingual area of the occlusion rim. The additional bulk of material is important for strength on the distal extension areas. A laboratory scalpel is used to clear the facial areas of the acrylic resin around the brass replicas and impression copings, exposing their interface. This interface is used to verify complete seating of the occlusion rim during maxillomandibular relations. When the acrylic resin record base has completely polymerized, it is carefully separated from the cast, and the relief wax is removed with a laboratory knife. The interface between the brass replica and the gold cylinder is opened for visualization on the facial surfaces. The borders of the record base are trimmed and polished (Fig. 3-26). The record base is placed on the working cast, guide pins are reinserted, and accuracy of the abutment coping interface is verified (Fig. 3-27). Baseplate wax is used to fabricate the occlusion rim in the usual fashion (Fig. 3-28). The mandibular occlusion rim can be fabricated initially to average dimensions (18 mm high anteriorly by 8 mm wide posteriorly). Access to each of the guide pins is created through the surface of the wax rim. The guide pins can be modified, either at this stage or by the restorative dentist, when the maxillomandibular relations are recorded. This is done so that the guide pins do not interfere with recording the correct occlusal vertical dimension and centric relation. The edges of the wax are finished to create smooth surfaces, and the accuracy of the interface between the coping and replica is rechecked (Fig. 3-29).

Clinical

Maxillomandibular Relations

The transitional dentures have established esthetics, phonetics, and temporomandibular joint response to the established vertical dimension of occlusion. The patient's response to the established patterns of the interim prosthesis are used as a guide for contouring wax rims and establishing vertical dimension. The mandibular occlusion rim is stabilized with either gold copings or altered impression copings (Fig. 3-30). Centric relation records, protrusive records, and a facebow registration are made (Fig. 3-31). At this appointment, tooth shade and denture tooth mold are selected, and the occlusal scheme is selected, depending on the nature of the maxillary arch and its relationship with the mandible.

Esthetic Trial Fitting

The casts are mounted on a semiadjustable articulator, using the facebow and centric relation records. The protrusive record is used for setting the condylar inclination. The wax occlusion rims are used as a guide for setting the denture teeth. Anterior (Figs. 3-32 and 3-33) and full tooth trial fittings are used to establish esthetics, phonetics, lip support, and the proper vertical dimension of occlusion. Centric relation is also verified with the interocclusal records.

The maximum distal extension cantilever is 15 mm distal to the distal-most, fixture abutment unit bilaterally. The distance is modified by the following factors:

1. Arch form of fixture abutment units

Fixture placement in a straight line places more load on the fixtures, abutments, abutment screws, and all components than does placement with an arch form. Cantiliver is shortened to the equivalent of 10 mm.

2. Fixture length and prognosis

Distal fixtures shorter than 10 mm (or those placed in less-than-ideal bone) limit load potential, and cantiliver extension is shortened to the equivalent of 10 mm.

3. Anterior cantilever

Class II jaw relationships and lingual fixture placement may necessitate an anterior cantilever for proper tooth arrangement. Three separate cantilevered sections may be necessary for proper tooth arrangement. This increases the load on all fixtures and prosthetic components. The distal cantilever should be shortened in this situation.

4. Natural maxillary dentition

Natural maxillary dentition opposing the implant prosthesis applies more load to the mandibular prosthesis, and cantilevers should be shortened to 10 mm.

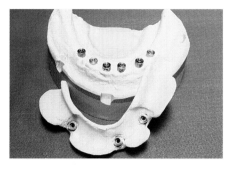

Fig. 3-26

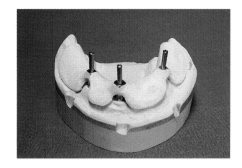

Fig. 3-27

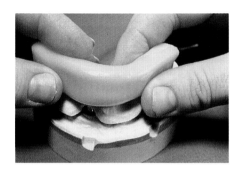

Fig. 3-28

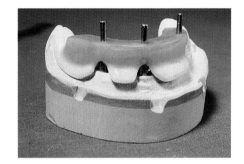

Fig. 3-29

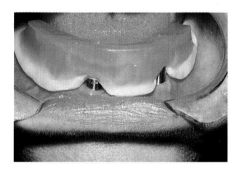

Fig. 3-30

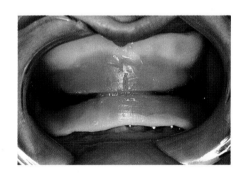

Fig. 3-31

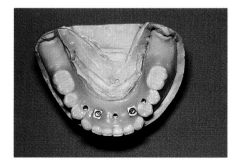

Fig. 3-32

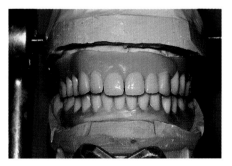

Fig. 3-33

5. Parafunctional habits

Clenching and bruxism add an additional load to fixtures and prosthetic components. Shortening distal cantilevers and fabrication of a nightguard will lessen the load on components. Before the framework is designed, the surgeon and the restorative dentist should discuss and record the fixture length and the quality of bone at the fixture placement. Other parameters are evaluated, and the final cantilever distances are used during tooth trial fittings and discussed with the dental technician for framework design. Excess cantilevers overload the fixtures and components. Possible consequences of overload include fixture loss and component loosening and fracture. (See complications in Chapter X.)

Laboratory

A survey of the master cast establishes the parameters used to determine both the symmetry and maximal extension of the distal portion of the implant-retained prosthesis (Figs. 3-34 and 3-35). It is believed that cantilevering the distal pontic area in excess of 10 mm in the maxillary arch and/or 15 mm in the mandibular arch beyond the terminal fixture will place excessive forces on the abutment fixtures. The functional force exerted on this area may be beyond the capacity of the osseointegrated fixtures to withstand. The result may include loss of fixtures and/or fracture of the prosthesis. Abutment and gold screws may loosen or fracture also.

To determine the maximal distal extension of the implant prosthesis, transfer the midline of the prosthesis to the master cast. The distance from the midline is measured to the most posterior left and right fixtures and is then recorded. The shortest measurement is used and added to the maximum allowable extension. This calculation is the maximum limit of the cantilever section of the implant prosthesis; however, the proposed tooth setup and type of occlusion that is to be developed may modify the cantilever length. The distance from the midline to the right distal fixture is 24 mm, and the distance from the midline to the left fixture is 28 mm. Measurements are made from the center of the abutment over the arch to the distal fixture. For example, in Fig. 3-34 the distance to the right distal abutment is the shortest; thus 15 mm are added to this distance to arrive at a maximum posterior extension of 39 mm from midline. Both sides are made no longer than the calculated measurement to keep the prosthesis symmetrical. These measurements must be accurate and are critical to the prosthesis distal extension strength.

After the preliminary denture setup has been completed, it is necessary to drill a vertical hole through selective denture teeth to gain access to the underlying fixture. The baseplate wax is removed from underneath the denture tooth, and the alignment of the fixture is determined by using the guide pin. A #10 round bur mounted in a straight handpiece is used to create a vertical access opening in the denture tooth, or the wax baseplate, to expose the brass replica (Fig. 3-36 and 3-37).

Clinical—Esthetic Trial Fitting

The completed prosthetic setup is returned to the clinic for an esthetic trial fitting (Fig. 3-38). All maxillomandibular relations are reverified and the occlusal contacts reconfirmed at this session (Fig. 3-39). The setup is returned to the dental laboratory where the construction of the framework will begin.

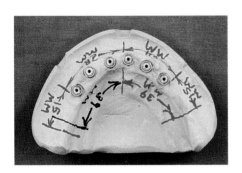

Fig. 3-34

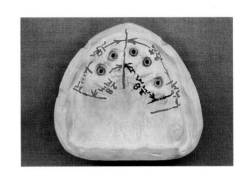

Fig. 3-35

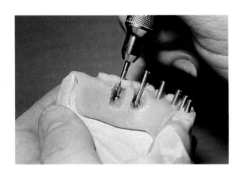

Fig. 3-36

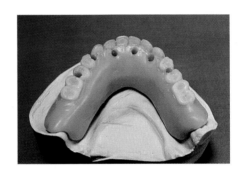

Fig. 3-37

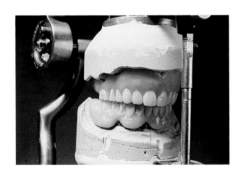

Fig. 3-38

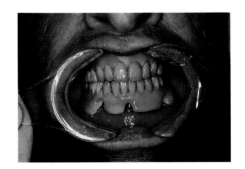

Fig. 3-39

Matrix Fabrication

A vinyl polysiloxane elastomer or laboratory plaster matrix is fabricated on the trial tooth setup to preserve the relationship of the teeth and waxing to the underlying cast framework.

The superior portion of the cast base is indexed in the following three areas: the anterior midline, the right posterior molar regions, and the left posterior molar region (Fig. 3-40). A grinding wheel mounted on a low-speed dental handpiece is used to complete this procedure. Indexing the cast in three diverse areas ensures that the matrix can be replaced on the cast in a firm, predictable position. The interproximal areas between the denture teeth are opened, using a wax carving instrument (Fig. 3-41). This allows the matrix material to flow readily between the teeth. It also makes it easier to position and hold the denture teeth in the matrix for repositioning on the framework. The vinyl polysiloxane elastomer of medium viscosity is mixed according to the manufacturer's directions and in sufficient quantity to be placed around the buccal and the labial and over the occlusal aspect of the denture setup. When the material is ready, it is molded across the anterior labial and the posterior buccal surfaces of the setup, forcing the material between the interproximal areas and into the indexing grooves on the cast base (Fig. 3-42). The material is worked across the teeth and around the guide pins. The completed matrix has impression material molded on all sides of the denture wax-up and the guide pins; only the tips of the guide pins are left exposed (Fig. 3-43). This procedure creates a positive orientation between cast and wax-up. A sectional plaster matrix is an alternative technique. The matrix is removed from the master cast, and the excess impression material is trimmed from the lingual surface of the wax-up, using a laboratory scalpel (Fig. 3-44). This area is removed from both the anterior and posterior lingual surfaces to give full access to the lingual surfaces during subsequent waxing procedures. The notched areas provide the positive orientation of the cast on the labial aspect of the impression material. The denture teeth are carefully removed from the tooth arrangement (Fig. 3-45). Any wax residue is removed with boiling water and then flushed with a mild detergent. The teeth are rinsed and dried before replacing them in the matrix. All the individual denture teeth are replaced into the matrix and held in place with a dab of sticky wax that is placed on a cusp tip or an incisal edge. The wax must be kept away from the guide pin holes. The matrix is placed back on the master cast when the teeth have been secured (Fig. 3-46). Adequate clearance between the guide pins and the denture teeth is verified.

Framework Wax-up

The implant components used in the framework waxing procedure are the guide pin, gold cylinder and screw, and the brass replica/analogue (Fig. 3-47). To stabilize the gold cylinders and minimize warpage of the wax pattern, a verification splint may be fabricated. When using the fine grained resin, make cuts between several sections, replace them on the cast, and recure them with new material to minimize internal stress. The substructure waxing is replaced on the master cast and secured with guide pins. The area below and around the abutment analogues is blocked out with modeling compound. Modeling compound is extended distally to the predetermined maximum extensions of the prosthesis framework. A small trough is created at the distal extension areas to be used as a receptacle for wax; the trough will control the flow of the wax and minimize the amount of wax used (Fig. 3-48). A wax separating medium is applied to the denture teeth within the matrix; this facilitates removal of the teeth from the framework waxing. The wax portion of the framework is fabricated quickly by luting the matrix to the cast with sticky wax or cyanoacrylate adhesive (Fig. 3-49). The gold cylinders, matrix, and splint are stablilized with the long lubri-

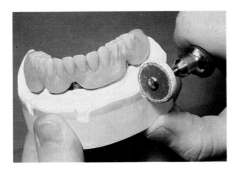

Fig. 3-40

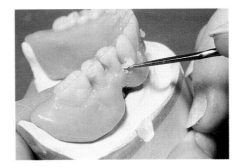

Fig. 3-41

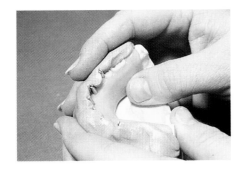

Fig. 3-42

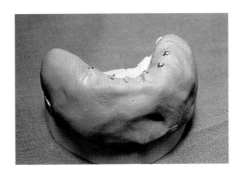

Fig. 3-43

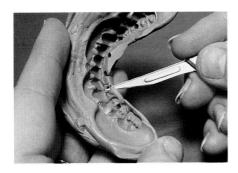

Fig. 3-44

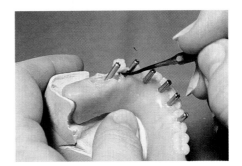

Fig. 3-45

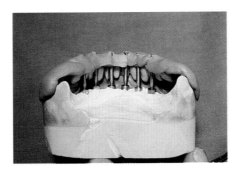

Fig. 3-46

cated guide pins. A glass eyedropper is filled with molten wax; the molten wax flows into the matrix over the luted denture teeth and the gold cylinders and then flows into the trough (Fig. 3-50). The wax is allowed to solidify at room temperature without applying any external coolant (Fig. 3-51). The waxing *must not* be chilled with cold water or cooled with compressed air because this may cause an internal stress formation within the wax pattern. The matrix is removed and any modeling compound is cleaned from the master cast and waxing (Fig. 3-52). The waxing is replaced on the master cast, and a reference line is placed on the side of the master cast base for each denture tooth midline. The line will serve as a guide for placement of retentive struts that will not interfere with the resetting of denture teeth (Fig. 3-53).

Excess wax is cleared from around the gold cylinders and the distal extension areas of the waxing (Fig. 3-54 and 3-55). The labial and lingual interproximal areas are opened around each of the abutment replicas, and concave contours are carved around the gold cylinders to allow sufficient space for hygiene (Fig. 3-56). The lingual contour is carved to allow room for the tongue. Excessive contour may interfere with speech. *Caution:* when completing the wax-up, try to work with the pattern on the master cast as much as possible. Handling of the fragile wax pattern might cause distortion or breakage.

The cantilevered pontic area of the waxing is positioned directly distal to the last abutment and is connected to the last cylinder with a J-shaped connector. The shape of this portion of the wax-up is important because it contributes to the strength of the distal extension. *Excessive cutback beyond the J-section may lead to fracture of the framework.* The ideal dimension of this J-section is 4 mm wide × 6 mm high (24 square mm). The pontic, connected to the J-section (Fig. 3-57), is positioned 1 mm to 2 mm above the tissues of the posterior residual ridge to prevent tissue hyperplasia and to allow room for adequate hygene procedures (Fig. 3-58). The wax is smoothed and sealed around the gold cylinders. This is achieved by lightly polishing the waxing with a cotton tipped applicator moistened with Xylene (Fig. 3-59). Any wax residue from the inferior surface of the gold cylinders must be removed, otherwise there may be casting flash over these areas. Xylene is used sparingly because it is a powerful solvent. It is used because it produces an even, smooth texture to the wax pattern (Fig. 3-60). After the complete waxing has been smoothed, the lingual surface of each distal extension section is marked for a wax cutback. A metal/acrylic resin finishing line is created halfway between the occlusal surface and the inferior border of the distal cantilevered section. The prosthesis waxing should be cut back one half of that distance. There are many different configurations to the lingual surface of the implant prosthesis wax-up, but the overriding consideration should be one of maintaining the strength of the casting. In the anterior lingual region, the metal/acrylic resin finishing line is designed anterior to the placement of the guide pins; this facilitates the procedure because it allows screw access in metal when removing the prosthesis at a later date (Fig. 3-61). On the labial and buccal surfaces a 1 to 2 mm finishing line is carved above the gold cylinders (Fig. 3-62). The wax pattern is hollowed out with a bur to provide maximum room for retention of the acrylic resin (Fig. 3-63). The interproximal areas are scalloped to allow a minimal amount of metal to be visible on the labial surface. In the distal extension areas, a minimum 24 mm^2 of metal must be maintained. There are four methods of providing retention to the cutback wax pattern: (1) undercuts placed around the guide pins; (2) 18-gauge wax retention bar placement; (3) application of plastic retention beads; and (4) bonding agents. With the wax pattern placed on the master cast, the predetermined reference marks are used to place 18-gauge wax strips in a vertical correspondence to the midline of the denture teeth (Fig. 3-64). Plastic retentive beads are also placed on the internal surfaces of the wax pattern for additional retention. A tacky liquid should be used on the portions of the wax-up to receive plastic beads (Fig. 3-65) before they are applied.

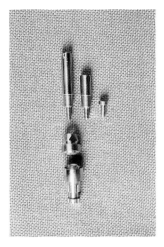

Fig. 3-47

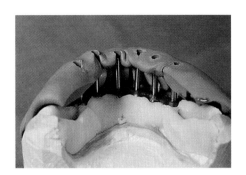

Fig. 3-48

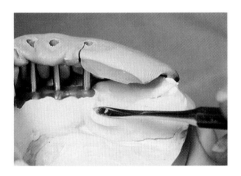

Fig. 3-49

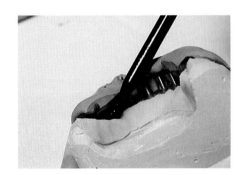

Fig. 3-50

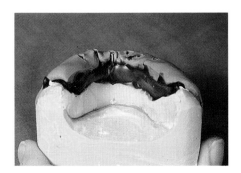

Fig. 3-51

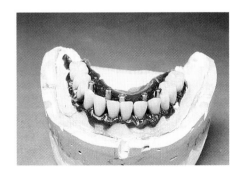

Fig. 3-52

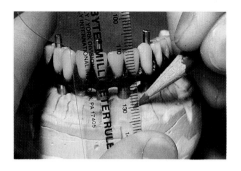

Fig. 3-53

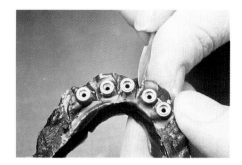

Fig. 3-54

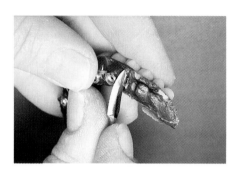

Fig. 3-55

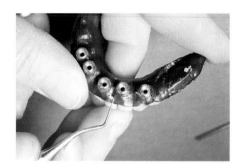

Fig. 3-56

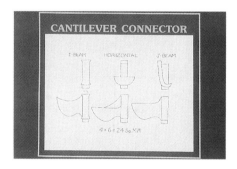

Fig. 3-57

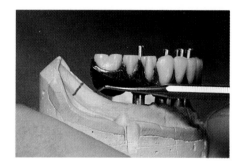

Fig. 3-58

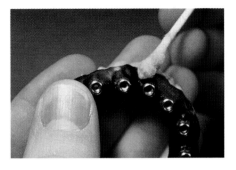

Fig. 3-59

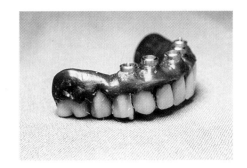

Fig. 3-60

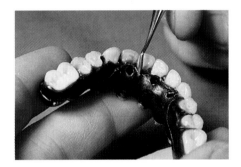

Fig. 3-61

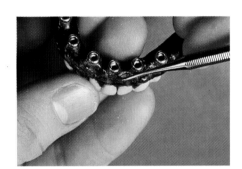

Fig. 3-62

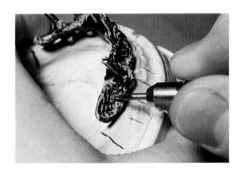

Fig. 3-63

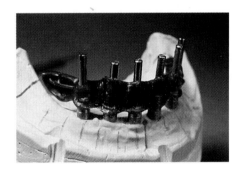

Fig. 3-64

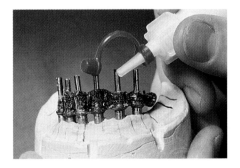

Fig. 3-65

Spruing

An indirect feeder bar spruing method is used in the casting of the prosthesis framework. A 6-gauge plastic feeder bar is heated, allowed to soften, and then bent to the arch form of the waxing (Fig. 3-66). The posterior ends are cross-stabilized with another piece of 6-guage plastic feeder bar (Fig. 3-67). Eight-gauge wax sprues that are 3 mm to 4 mm long are secured to the waxing between the guide pin holes, and two sprues are placed on each distal extension. A 6-gauge sprue is attached to the distal extension for cross-arch stabilization (Fig. 3-68). The size of the plastic feeder bar is determined by the bulky part of the waxing. The stabilized bar is coated with wax before it is attached to the sprues. Coating the bar with wax allows the wax to be eliminated through the sprue holes before the plastic bar is burned out and eliminates the entrapment of wax in the investment. Four 6-gauge auxiliary sprues are placed and angled indirectly for the attachment of the wax pattern to the sprue-former base (Fig. 3-69). The indirect spruing technique will ensure an even flow of molten alloy into the mold cavity. The completed sprued wax pattern is weighed to determine the amount of alloy necessary to complete the casting (Fig. 3-70). The wax pattern is placed on the sprue former, and a distal extension reference point is marked (Fig. 3-71 and 3-72). The gold cylinders are cleaned with an ammonia solution to remove any residual oil or other residue that might cause casting flash (Fig. 3-73). A casting ring of 400 to 600 grams in size is lined with a nonasbestos liner.

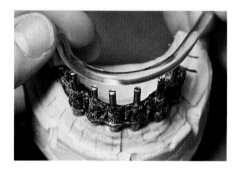

Fig. 3-66

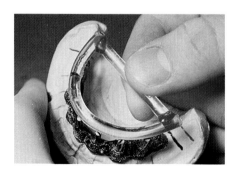

Fig. 3-67

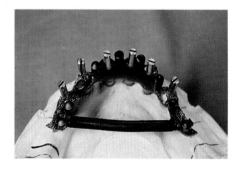

Fig. 3-68

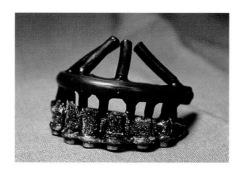

Fig. 3-69

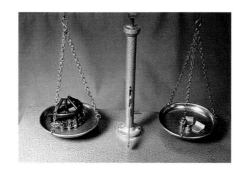

Fig. 3-70

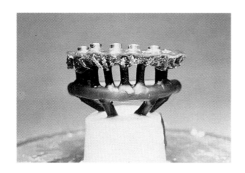

Fig. 3-71

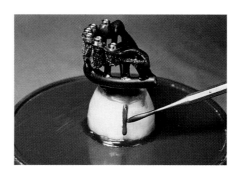

Fig. 3-72

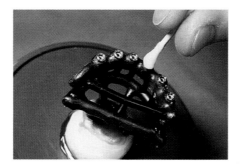

Fig. 3-73

Selecting the Casting Alloy

A variety of metals may be used to cast the framework: ceramic, gold, or palladium-silver alloys; however, the metal that is selected must meet a minimum tensile strength of 60,000 psi. In the United States the use of a palladium-silver alloy is preferred, primarily because of cost factors. The chosen alloy should be able to be cast at a temperature below 2,300° Fahrenheit (F). The gold cylinders will be damaged if the casting temperature is higher than 2,300° F. The method used to determine the amount of alloy needed to assure a complete casting is determined by the following formula:

$$\text{Wax weight} \times \text{Specific gravity} = \text{Amount of alloy needed}$$
$$(\text{e.g., } 3.75 \text{ DWT} \times 10.6 = 39.75 \text{ DWT})$$

The amount of metal required is governed by the specific gravity of the alloy and that is determined by the manufacturer. Using this formula reduces the costly error associated with using either too little or too much alloy for the casting.

Investing the Wax Pattern

Orient the waxing in the selected casting ring, leaving 10 mm to 13 mm of space all around the pattern for investment. Allow for at least 6 mm of investment over the top of the waxing (Fig. 3-74). The sprue-former base is marked to orient the distal extension portion of the pattern so that it can be correctly aligned in the cradle of the casting machine. When the ring is cast, it should be arranged in the centrifugal casting machine with the marked distal extensions in a trailing position. A high-heat, phosphate-bound investment is used with a powder/liquid ratio to achieve maximum expansion when palladium-silver alloy or other similar metal is cast. The investment is poured into the casting ring statically; the clinician must be careful not to entrap air in the guide pin holes because the investment must come up through the holes (Fig. 3-75).

Casting the Wax Pattern

A two-stage burnout system is recommended when using the large investment rings. When oxygen and natural gas are used, the oxygen pressure is set at 15 to 20 pounds, and the ring is cast after burnout in a normal fashion. Make sure the distal extension portion of the casting ring is placed in the trailing position of the machine's cradle.

Finishing the Casting

The casting is roughly broken out from the investment, and the clinician must be careful to protect the gold cylinders and the inferior surface of the casting. *Do not use any abrasives that will cause damage to either the inferior surfaces or the gold cylinders.* The casting is cleaned with aluminum oxide or glass beads, protecting the gold cylinders (Fig. 3-76 and 3-77). Protection caps placed over the cylinders will help to eliminate possible damage. The framework is removed from the feeder sprues and stabilizing bar, using a separating disc mounted on a low-speed handpiece (Fig. 3-78). A #10 round bur is used to remove investment from the guide pin holes, being careful not to damage the seat of the gold cylinders (Fig. 3-79 and 3-80). Damage to the gold cylinder seat will keep the prosthesis from seating accurately. After each guide pin hole has been cleaned, the casting is placed back on the master cast and checked circumferentially for interface accuracy between each brass replica and gold cylinder. Complete interface accuracy should be established with one guide pin screwed in

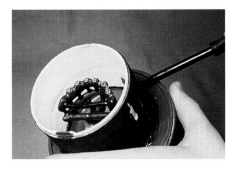

Fig. 3-74

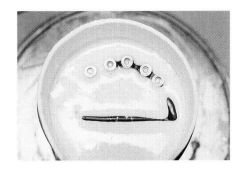

Fig. 3-75

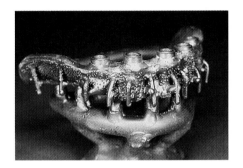

Fig. 3-76

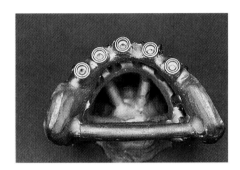

Fig. 3-77

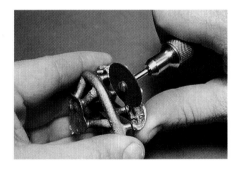

Fig. 3-78

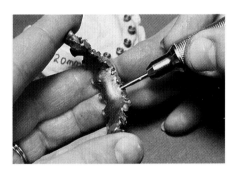

Fig. 3-79

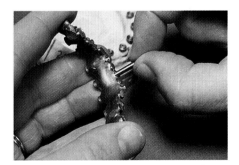

Fig. 3-80

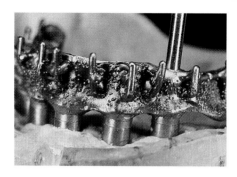

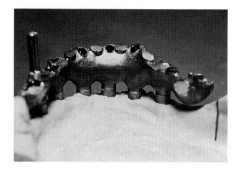

Fig. 3-81   Fig. 3-82

place anywhere on the casting (Fig. 3-81 and 3-82). The casting can then be returned to the clinic for a trial fitting.

Framework Trial Fitting

The abutments are thoroughly cleaned and the titanium hemostats and hexagonal wrench are used to confirm abutment tightness. The framework is tried on the abutments using only passive tightening of the gold alloy screws in an incremental tightening pattern (Fig. 3-83). The abutment framework-interface should show intimate and circumferential contact for all abutments. Tenderness during tightening may indicate improper fit. If pain is elicited at this time, it may indicate an ill-fitting framework. If the patient reports sensitivity in one of the distal fixtures, this may also indicate proximity to the mental nerve. A mirror must be used to check for intimate fit. If the interface inaccuracy is noticed, the framework must be sectioned around the ill-fitting segment. The framework is removed from the mouth and sectioned, using an ultrafine separating disc (Fig. 3-84). Care should be taken to keep the cut no greater than 0.4 mm for ease of soldering. The sectioned framework is tried in the mouth to ensure intimate fit between all abutments and the framework. The segments are aligned, making sure that there is no metal contact between sections.

The sections are luted while secured in the mouth with autopolymerizing resin (Fig. 3-85). This can be accomplished by filling a syringe with mixed resin and inserting the resin into each of the sectioned areas. A straight handpiece bur can be used to cross-arch stabilize the framework in the mouth. The resined framework is allowed to polymerize, the guide pins are removed, and the sectioned, resin-secured framework is returned to the laboratory for soldering.

Soldering

If the casting does not accurately fit the master cast as previously described or if it does not seat completely upon clinical trial fitting, the casting must be sectioned and the framework parts must be soldered together in the laboratory. Since the casting no longer fits the master cast, the cast is altered to fit the casting (Fig. 3-86). The brass replicas corresponding to the altered section of the framework are removed from the master cast with a separating disc (Figs. 3-87 through 3-89). Residual stone is removed from around each misaligned replica and replaced on the framework; the framework is then remounted with the guide pin screws on the master cast. Complete relief around each replica is verified (Fig. 3-90). A small portion of diestone is mixed and placed around the brass replicas (Fig. 3-91) and allowed to set. The autopolymerizing resin is removed from the casting by heating it over an open Bunsen burner flame. Each of the cleaned segments is replaced on this adjusted master cast.

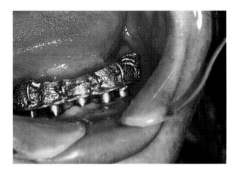

Fig. 3-83

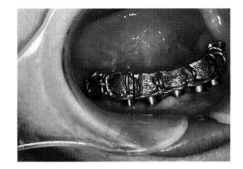

Fig. 3-84

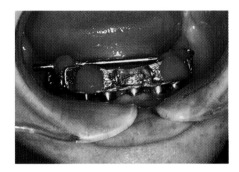

Fig. 3-85

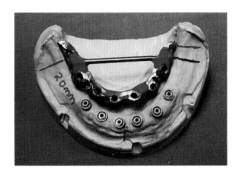

Fig. 3-86

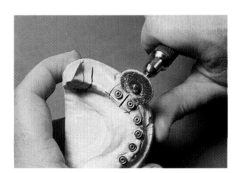

Fig. 3-87

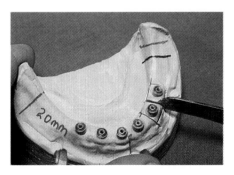

Fig. 3-88

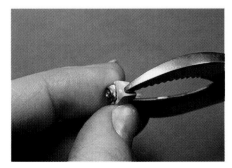

Fig. 3-89

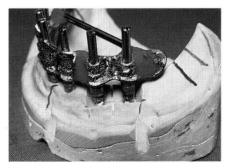

Fig. 3-90

To stabilize the framework segments, sticky wax is flowed into each joint place to be soldered, and a bar is placed across the arch to reach each solder joint (Fig. 3-92). The sticky wax is chilled by running the cast under cold water. Additional sticky wax is placed on the inferior surfaces of the solder joint areas. *Extreme care is made to not get sticky wax on the gold cylinder surface or interface, or solder will flash over these areas.* The framework is placed in soldering investment and allowed to set (Fig. 3-93). The sticky wax is removed by flushing the investment with boiling water; then the surfaces are cleaned with a detergent. The investment is relieved to provide access to the joints that are to be soldered (Fig. 3-94). Soldering flux is placed in the joint space, and the investment is preheated for an even expansion. When each joint is soldered, the investment is heated from the labial aspect, and solder is placed on the lingual surface and allowed to *pull through* from the lingual to the labial surface (Fig. 3-95). The soldered framework and investment are allowed to cool at room temperature. The casting is removed from the investment, cleaned, remounted on the altered master cast, and checked for the interface seating of the casting to the brass replicas.

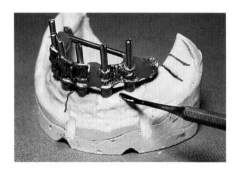

Fig. 3-91

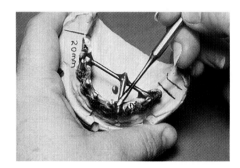

Fig. 3-92

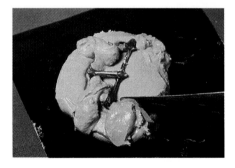

Fig. 3-93

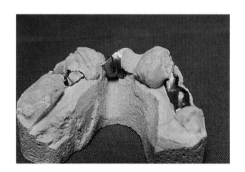

Fig. 3-94

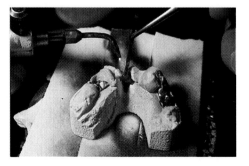

Fig. 3-95

Polishing the Framework

Before any abrasive cleaning or finishing of the casting is done, the gold cylinders should be protected with protection caps or altered brass replicas (Fig. 3-96). *Negligence in this area may cause damage to the interface surfaces* (Fig. 3-97). *This is one of the most critical steps in the prosthesis fabrication. Failure to protect the interface surfaces at this point will result in destroying the seat of the prosthesis.* The retentive area of the brass replica is removed, using a separating disc mounted in a low-speed handpiece (Fig. 3-98). This allows the dental technician to gain access to the undersurface and the interproximal areas of the framework to use a rubber wheel and polish the frame without damaging the gold cylinders. This protective measure should be used when cleaning with an air abrasive and finishing both the metal framework and the subsequent acrylic resin (Fig. 3-99). The final framework can be smoothed by using a number of different finishing methods and materials. Rubber wheels and/or points mounted in a low-speed handpiece are used to finish the framework (Fig. 3-100). The metal/acrylic resin finishing line is smoothed and finished, using a carbide bur mounted in a high-speed handpiece (Fig. 3-101). The final high shine is imparted to the framework, using a felt wheel and polishing compound. After the casting is finished and polished, it is ultrasonically cleaned and replaced on the working cast. Casting is returned to the clinic for trial fitting and interface verification (Fig. 3-102).

Clinical

The framework is again seated in the mouth passively, and the abutment framework interface is evaluated as previously described. Visual inspection is used to verify intimate 360-degree contact between all abutment framework interfaces. The screws are tightened, and the patient is asked to report any pain as the framework is tightened. Either a mechanical or electric torque wrench is used to tighten to 10 Ncm. If the interfaces are accurate and no pain is elicited, the framework is removed in preparation for adding denture teeth. If the framework is ill fitting, it is again sectioned, indexed, and soldered until accurate fit is achieved. The fit of the framework is crucial to the long-term success of the prosthesis; many problems can be caused by an ill-fitting framework (see Chapter 10).

Denture Tooth Waxing

The denture teeth are replaced into the vinyl polysiloxane matrix using sticky wax. The exact placement of the teeth is reconfirmed by comparing the tooth position with the reference marks placed on the side of the master cast.

Additional mechanical retention should be replaced in each denture tooth to ensure both a strong mechanical/chemical bonding of the denture tooth to the processed acrylic resin. Either a #2 or a #4 round bur mounted in a low-speed handpiece is used to drill small holes into the lingual surface of each denture tooth (Fig. 3-103). This is completed before the teeth are placed in the matrix. The matrix is replaced on the master cast containing the finished framework (Fig. 3-104). The denture teeth should not interfere with any of the retentive features (struts, beads). A glass eyedropper filled with molten baseplate wax is used to flow the molten wax between the teeth and casting incrementally, until the matrix is filled. The wax is allowed to solidify (Fig. 3-105). The matrix is removed and the areas around the denture teeth are carved and festooned. The occlusal contacts are verified with the casts on the articulator, and the prosthesis is returned to the clinic (Fig. 3-106).

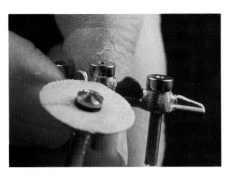

Fig. 3-96

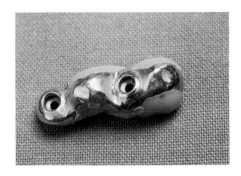

Fig. 3-97

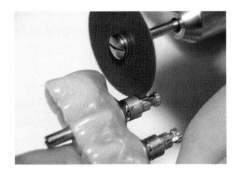

Fig. 3-98

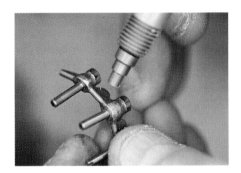

Fig. 3-99

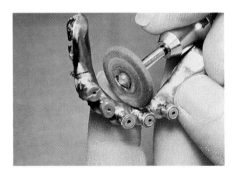

Fig. 3-100

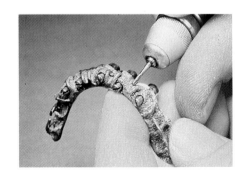

Fig. 3-101

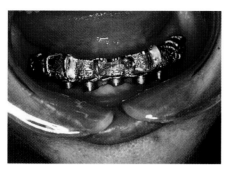

Fig. 3-102

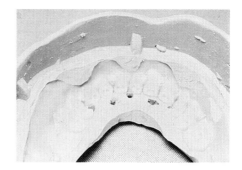

Fig. 3-103

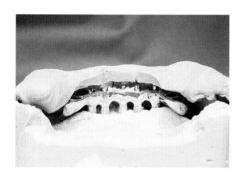

Fig. 3-104

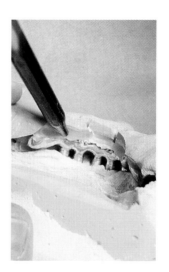

Fig. 3-105

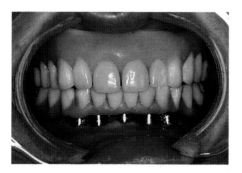

Fig. 3-106

Clinical—Full Trial Tooth Arrangement on Framework

The full trial tooth arrangement on the maxillary occlusion rim and the mandibular framework is assessed in a final evaluation of all maxillomandibular relations. The patient is asked to closely evaluate the esthetics before the processing of the prostheses. At this time it may be helpful to have a family member or personal friend of the patient evaluate the esthetics also. After the patient approves the prosthesis, a centric relation record is made, and the prosthesis is ready for processing.

Laboratory—Acrylic Processing and Final Finishing the Framework

Three methods are used in processing the denture teeth to the framework: (1) conventional trial packing and processing; (2) injection mold processing; and (3) light-cured composite processing. (Because of the complex steps that ensure total polymerization of the light-cured resin, along with the labor intensity to hand layer and manipulate the material before processing, it is not a preferred method.) The conventional trial packing method is adequate, but problems may arise if the guide pins are not parallel; as a result, trial packing may have to be eliminated (Figs. 3-107 through 3-109). The injection mold processing, such as Ivoclar (Ivocap system), is the most desirable. Because the denture material is injected and cured under high pressure, the acrylic is denser and hyperocclusion problems are eliminated.

To minimize processing changes that may occur, the processing of the acrylic resin is done while the prosthesis waxing is seated on the master cast.

The prosthesis and master cast are invested in the bottom half of a denture flask (Fig. 3-110), and then the rest of the flasking procedure is completed in a normal method (Fig. 3-111). The flask is placed in a boilout tank, is heated, and the wax is removed (Fig. 3-112). Both halves of the denture flask, mold cavity, and denture teeth are scrubbed, cleaned, and allowed to cool. A bonding agent may be applied to the frame to enhance the bond between the acrylic and the metal. Bonding agent *must not* be applied to the exposed area of the guide pins, or the guide pins will become permanently bonded. It is also recommended to apply a tissue tinted opaque to mask out the shadowy effect of the cast frame, which will cause the final processed acrylic to be dark.

The prosthesis is processed in a high-impact acrylic resin, using a standard curing cycle that is recommended by the manufacturer (Fig. 3-113). The prosthesis is carefully removed from the flask. A laboratory remount and occlusal adjustment are completed. It may be necessary to use a soldering iron to lightly heat each guide pin to remove it from the prosthesis (Figs. 3-114 and 3-115).

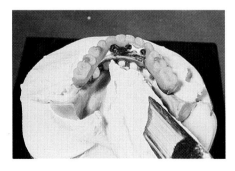

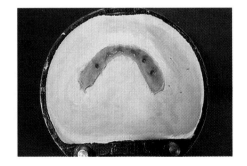

Fig. 3-107   Fig. 3-108

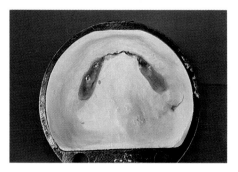

Fig. 3-109

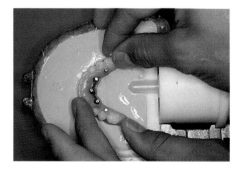

Fig. 3-110

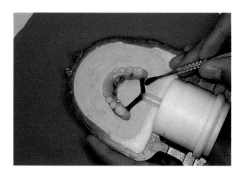

Fig. 3-111

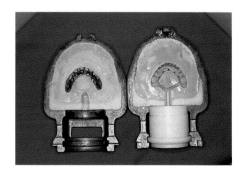

Fig. 3-112

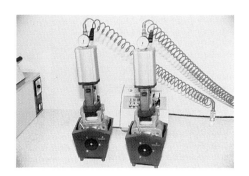

Fig. 3-113

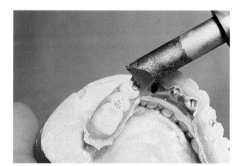

Fig. 3-114

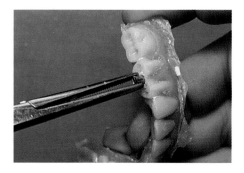

Fig. 3-115

The final casting can be smoothed with a number of different finishing methods and materials, but continued practice of extreme caution should be taken to protect the gold cylinders from damage during any finishing procedures. Protection caps or brass analogues are placed over the gold cylinders and the prosthesis is finished and polished, using rubber points, wheels, and pumice (Fig. 3-116). A rag wheel with polishing compound is used to give the implant prosthesis its final luster (Fig. 3-117). Soap and water and/or an ultrasonic bath are used to clean residual polishing materials from the prosthesis. The prosthesis is replaced on the master cast and the interface between the gold cylinders and abutment replicas is reverified.

Clinical Delivery

The patient is instructed to leave out the existing maxillary denture for several hours before the implant prosthesis is inserted, if applicable. The maxillary denture is checked with a pressure indicator paste in the usual method. A centric relation record is made with both prostheses in position (Figs. 3-118 through 3-122). A laboratory remount is completed. The occlusion is then refined in the mouth, using articulating paper and shimstock. The gold screws are tightened with one of the torque wrenches, and temporary fillings are placed in the screw access holes (Figs. 3-123 and 3-124). The patient then is seen by the hygienist for homecare instructions.

The patient returns to the clinic the following day, and the restorative dentist rechecks the tightness of the screws and discusses any complications that may have occurred overnight with the patient. The patient is scheduled for another recall in one week, and the same checks are made. The prosthesis will be permanently seated at the 1-month recall. The patient then is scheduled for recall at 6 months, depending on oral hygiene skills.

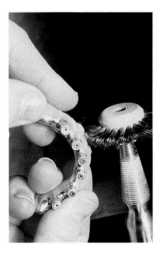

Fig. 3-116

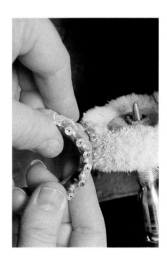

Fig. 3-117

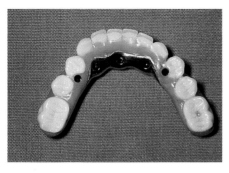

Fig. 3-118

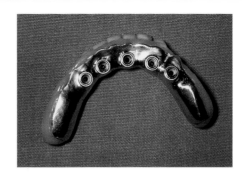

Fig. 3-119

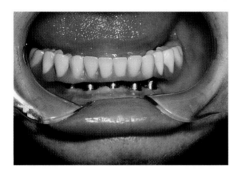

Fig. 3-120

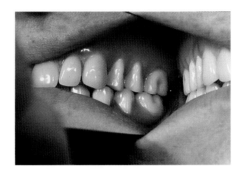

Fig. 3-121

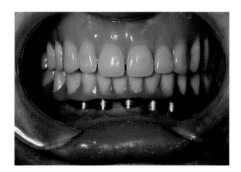

Fig. 3-122

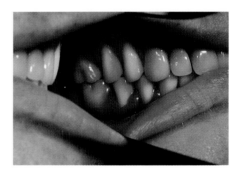

Fig. 3-123

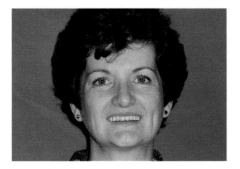

Fig. 3-124

4

Completely Edentulous Fixed Implant-Retained Prosthesis—Maxillary Arch

The esthetic demands in the maxillary arch may dictate the type of implant-retained prosthesis. When a patient comes to the restorative dentist for consultation for a tissue-integrated prosthesis in the maxilla, the patient's desires and expectations must be explored. Models of different prosthetic options are shown, including full contour overdenture, overdenture with the palate removed, and the completely edentulous fixed prosthesis. Photographs of patients who have completed treatment are useful, also. After the patient is interviewed, a clinical examination is completed. The existing dentures are evaluated for lip support, vertical dimension of occlusion, retention, and esthetics, including the height of smile line. The labial flange thickness of the maxillary denture is measured, and the patient is questioned concerning his or her satisfaction with lip support (Figs. 4-1 through 4-4). The distal-most tooth that shows during maximum smile is recorded, also. A smile line that reveals first or second molars may cause an esthetic compromise because of cantilever restrictions for an implant prosthesis in the maxilla (Fig. 4-5). *The patient should be involved in these observations and should communicate his or her expectations to the restorative dentist.* The patient may have definite desires and may prefer an overdenture or a fixed prosthesis. *No commitment for the type of maxillary prosthesis should be indicated by the restorative dentist at this time.*

Surgical Evaluation

The surgeon and the restorative dentist should consult after the patient's surgical evaluation. For an implant prosthesis in the maxilla, a minimum of five fixtures is needed. If the location and amount of bone are adequate for five fixtures, the possibility of an implant prosthesis can be explored with the patient during a second consultation appointment. If the bone is inadequate for five fixtures or if the contours are inadequate for lip support, an overdenture is the treatment of choice. If the patient still desires an implant-retained fixed prosthesis, bone grafting may be an option (see Chapter 8).

The factors affecting prosthetic success are discussed with the patient. Limitations in the posterior tooth extension and compromise in esthetics from lack of tissue support, both labially and buccally, are explored. The transition from complete palatal coverage to an implant prosthesis requires adjustment and compensation by the tongue to changed morphology in the oral cavity. Fixture placement and frame-

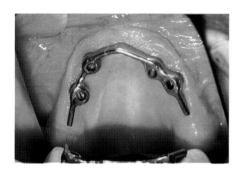

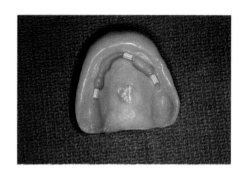

Fig. 4-1

Fig. 4-2

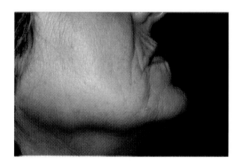

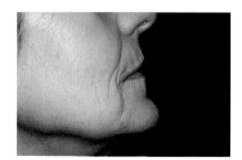

Fig. 4-3

Fig. 4-4

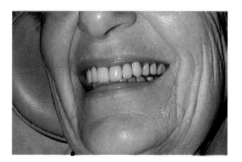

Fig. 4-5

work position affect articulation, and speech may be altered for 1 to 6 months. The patient must be made aware of potential speech difficulties. If no speech problems exist with a complete denture, the patient will adapt, and speech will return to normal after approximately 1 month with the fixed prosthesis.

The patient's dexterity and motivation for hygiene protocol must be assessed. The fixed prosthesis requires dexterity and motivation for optimum maintenance (see Chapter 10). After the consultations, *the patient who desires an implant prosthesis should be advised that the prosthetic design cannot be determined until after the abutment surgery and the diagnostic appointments are completed.* Fabrication of a transitional prosthesis or a treatment denture is completed before surgery. Traditional techniques and materials are used to establish an acceptable esthetic, phonetic, and functional removable prosthesis at the proper vertical dimension of occlusion. This allows elimination of unhealthy oral tissues from an ill-fitting prosthesis. Temporomandibular joint response to the vertical dimension of occlusion may be evaluated also. Lip support is established by the denture flange thickness labially, and indicates whether acceptable esthetics may be accomplished with a fixed prosthesis. After the transitional denture is completed, planning for fixture placement can begin.

Clinical and Laboratory Prosthetic Procedures
Diagnostic/Surgical Stent

The transitional maxillary denture is used as a guide for the surgical stent. The denture is duplicated and modified. See previously documented fabrication procedures of the diagnostic and surgical stents.

Tissue Treatment After Surgery

In patients who do not have bone grafts, the transitional denture is relieved in the surgical site, and the tissue conditioning material is placed in the denture 7 to 10 days after surgery and suture removal (Figs. 4-6 and 4-7). The patient occludes lightly, while the tissue conditioner sets. After the initial set (approximately 8 to 10 minutes), the denture is placed in a pressure pot at 20 psi for 10 minutes. The tissue conditioner lining is replaced as the patient heals, and the denture is relined after complete healing: 1½ to 2 months after surgery.

Patients who have had bone grafts are placed on a soft diet for 1 month after surgery and do not use a prosthesis. Usually a new denture must be made at this time because the graft will have drastically changed the maxillary morphology.

Tissue treatment material also is placed in the relieved prosthesis after second stage surgery. The healing caps are left on the abutments while the tissue treatment reline is made. The prosthesis has increased retention and stability following this procedure.

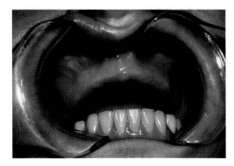

Fig. 4-6

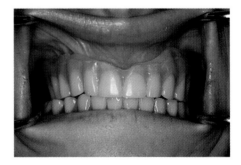

Fig. 4-7

Branemark Transmucosal Abutment

The prosthetic components used with the Branemark implant system have a long history of excellence in conjunction with patient rehabilitation. The Branemark system components include the titanium fixture, which is surgically placed in bone and remains submerged below the mucoperiosteum for 6 to 8 months in the maxilla while the osseointegration occurs. The titanium transmucosal abutment is placed on the implant during the second surgical procedure (Figs. 4-8 and 4-9). Transmucosal abutments are available in several lengths to accommodate prosthetic procedures and to allow the abutment to be placed 1 mm to 2 mm above the mucoperiosteum. The gold alloy cylinder, which is available in 3 mm and 4 mm heights, is incorporated into the framework. The gold screw is used to fix the cylinder, framework, and prosthesis unit to the transmucosal abutments and fixtures. These components are satisfactory for most implant-retained prostheses.

Preliminary Impression Procedures

Stock edentulous alginate trays are used to make the maxillary impression 10 to 20 days after the abutment surgery (Fig. 4-10). The cast will show the position of the transmucosal abutments in preparation for the custom tray fabrication.

Custom Tray Fabrication

The custom tray for the maxillary implant-retained prosthesis is fabricated in the same manner as previously documented for the mandible.

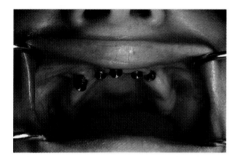

Fig. 4-8

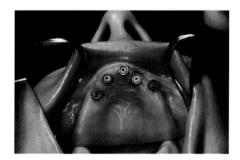

Fig. 4-9

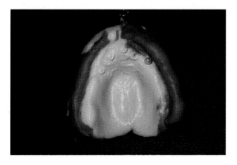

Fig. 4-10

Final Impressions

The healing caps are removed, and the hexagonal wrench and titanium hemostats are used to check abutment tightness. This procedure should be done at the beginning of every prosthetic appointment. All plaque and calculus are removed, and the impression copings are seated (Fig. 4-11). The custom tray is tried in the mouth and is adjusted for path of insertion (Fig. 4-12). The window for the tray then is covered with one thickness of baseplate wax, and the edges are sealed with a hot wax spatula (Fig. 4-13). The tray is heated in a water bath and is reseated in the mouth to capture the guide pin relationship (Fig. 4-14). After the adhesive is placed (Fig. 4-15), a medium viscosity vinyl polysiloxane or other appropriate impression material is mixed according to the manufacturer's directions. A 50 ml syringe and the impression tray are loaded, and the tray is seated in the mouth allowing the guide pins to penetrate the preformed wax holes (Fig. 4-16). The tray is held in position, while border molding is completed. After the impression material has set, the guide pins are loosened, and the impression is removed (Fig. 4-17). Laboratory analogues are placed (Fig. 4-18), and the impression is poured in die stone as previously described.

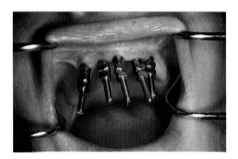

Fig. 4-11

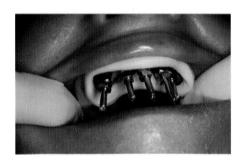

Fig. 4-12

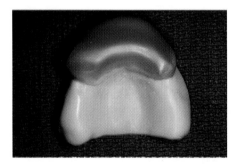

Fig. 4-13

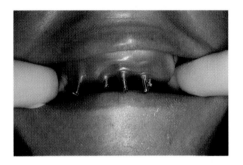

Fig. 4-14

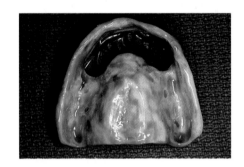

Fig. 4-15

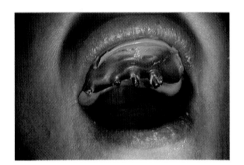

Fig. 4-16

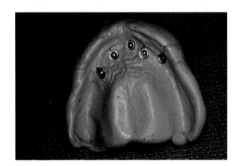

Fig. 4-17

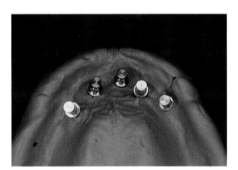

Fig. 4-18

Maxillomandibular Relations

Maxillomandibular relations are recorded, using a customized record base and interocclusion wax rim (Figs. 4-19 through 4-21). These are fabricated in a similar fashion as previously described. Gold cylinders or altered impression copings allow the securing of the record base to the transmucosal abutments for accurate interocclusal records. The wax rims are contoured to establish lip support, incisal edge position, buccal corridor, and midline and vertical dimensions of occlusion. Phonetics and other parameters that are employed in conventional denture techniques are also used. Centric relation, eccentric records, a facebow registration, tooth selection, and occlusal scheme are all made by the restorative dentist at this time.

The master and opposing casts are mounted on a semiadjustable articulator. The eccentric records are used for the articulator settings. The master cast is surveyed, and a full upper denture setup is completed by the laboratory.

Anterior and Full Esthetic Trial Fitting

These appointments are used to establish tooth position in regard to esthetics, phonetics, and vertical dimension of occlusion (Figs. 4-22 and 4-23). The transitional denture is used as a guide if the esthetics of the prosthesis are acceptable to the patient and to the restorative dentist. When the esthetics have been approved, the laboratory technician has the guidelines for framework fabrication.

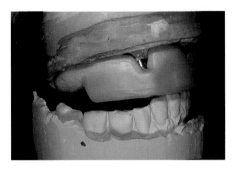

Fig. 4-19

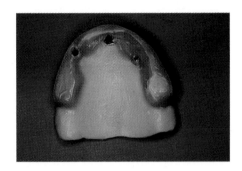

Fig. 4-20

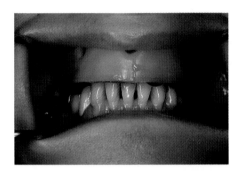

Fig. 4-21

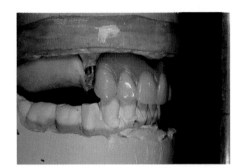

Fig. 4-22

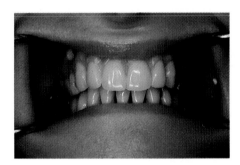

Fig. 4-23

Framework Fabrication

The framework fabrication for the maxillary implant-retained prosthesis is similar to that for the mandibular prosthesis. The esthetic denture trial fitting is used to establish the relationship of the framework to the final prosthesis. The matrix is fabricated in the same manner as previously stated in Chapter 3. The gold cylinders are placed on the master cast with guide pins (Fig. 4-24). The master cast is blocked out with compound, the guide pins are lubricated, and the matrix is reorientated to the master cast and held in place with sticky wax (Fig. 4-25). The matrix is filled with molten inlay wax and is allowed to solidify (Fig. 4-26). The matrix is removed, and the full contoured waxing is completed (Fig. 4-27). Proper periocontours must be incorporated into the framework design of the implant prosthesis. Ideally, convex surfaces are more desirable for an implant prosthesis, but in the maxilla, along with problems of bone resorption, a compromise may have to be made to maintain esthetic lip support. Cutback is performed and retention is provided for final processing of the denture base resin and for placement of teeth (Fig. 4-28). The wax pattern is indirectly sprued, invested, cast, reclaimed, and replaced on the master cast for fit verification (Figs. 4-29 through 4-31).

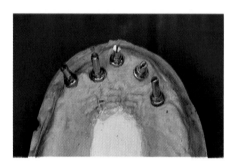

Fig. 4-24

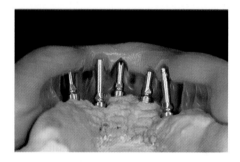

Fig. 4-25

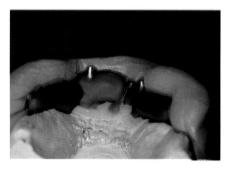

Fig. 4-26

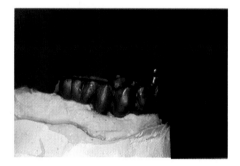

Fig. 4-27

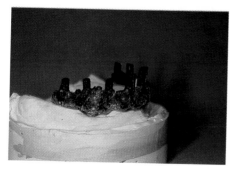

Fig. 4-28

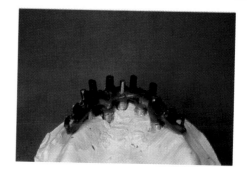

Fig. 4-29

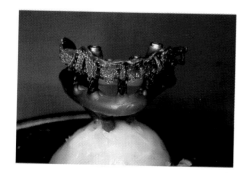

Fig. 4-30

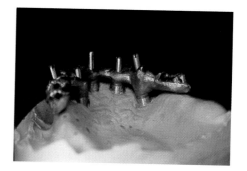

Fig. 4-31

Clinical—Framework Trial Fitting

The healing caps are removed, abutments cleaned and tightened, and the framework is seated passively with guide pins or gold screws (Figs. 4-32 and 4-33). Each abutment framework interface is checked circumferentially for intimacy of fit. Mirror views are used for verification of the palatal interface. Any discrepancy in the interface requires that the framework be sectioned, reverifying fit and solder indexing as seen previously in the mandibular section of Chapter 3.

The framework is reverified if soldering is necessary. Another indication that the framework may be inaccurate occurs when the patient experiences sensitivity during the tightening of screws. If sensitivity persists during several attempts at sequential slow tightening of the gold screws, then the framework in the area of this fixture must be sectioned, and a new solder index is made.

Full Esthetic Trial Fitting

The index used for framework waxing is used as a guide for resetting teeth on the frame. Esthetics and other parameters are verified again, and a centric relation record is made (Fig. 4-34). Adjustable mirrors may be useful in verifying esthetics. Lateral views are beneficial for patient verification of lip and tissue support. A friend or relative may be helpful at the full tooth arrangement appointment, when the patient makes a final decision about the esthetics of the arrangement.

Laboratory—Processing and Finishing

The laboratory processing and finishing procedures are performed for the maxillary implant prosthesis in the same manner as previously documented for the mandible. The finished prosthesis is returned to the clinic for delivery to the patient (Figs. 4-35 and 4-36).

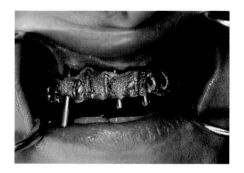

Fig. 4-32

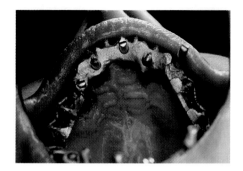

Fig. 4-33

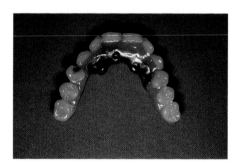

Fig. 4-34

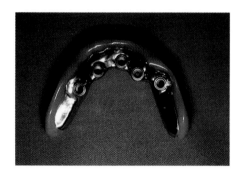

Fig. 4-35

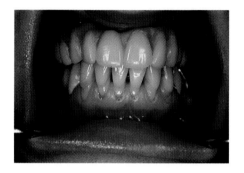

Fig. 4-36

Clinical Delivery

The healing caps are removed, the abutments are cleaned and tightened, and the prosthesis is seated (Figs. 4-37 through 4-41). The gold screws are sequentially tightened using the torque wrench for final tightness (Fig. 4-42). Occlusion is checked with occlusal ribbon and shimstock. If occlusal discrepancies have occurred during framework processing, a laboratory remount will be required. Cotton pellets and a temporary filling material are placed in the screw access holes. The patient then is seen by the hygienist for home care instructions and hygiene armamentarium. The patient is scheduled for recalls as described previously. Final filling is done as previously described.

◆ MAXILLARY COMBINATION COMPOSITE/PORCELAIN OCCLUSION

Patients with minimal maxillary resorption or those having had bone grafts may have minimal room for denture teeth set on a metal framework. Prosthesis design in these situations is best accomplished using a framework with porcelain veneer similar to a traditional fixed partial denture. The decision on whether to use the hybrid prosthesis with denture teeth or the porcelain fused to metal prosthesis is determined during complete trial fitting appointments (Fig. 4-43). Minimal room to retain denture teeth indicates that use of the porcelain fused to metal prosthesis is necessary. A high smile line may cause esthetic and hygienic compromise if the hybrid prosthesis is used (Figs. 4-44 and 4-45). Ridge lap porcelain pontics supported by the implant framework may be more esthetic and more accessible for cleaning (Figs. 4-46 and 4-47). The pioneering Swedish implant teams used porcelain fused to metal restorations, as well as resin systems; they found higher incidence of fixture loss with the porcelain fused to metal prostheses, and therefore recommended using the resin systems for esthetic veneering. A dampening effect from the resin during mastication and parafunctional activities was indicated as a positive influence on preserving osseointegration. Resin has the disadvantage of being less esthetic than porcelain and may intrinsically stain. A combination prosthesis has been developed that retains the advantages of both veneering methods. The framework has porcelain applied on the buccal surface to a 1 mm metal finish line on the palatal slope of the buccal cusps (Figs. 4-48 and 4-49). Light-cured composite is used on the occlusal surface of posterior teeth in all areas of occlusal contact. Therefore, the esthetics of porcelain are combined with the dampening effect and wear pattern of the composite resin (Fig. 4-50).

Clinical

Impression technique, maxillomandibular relations, and trial fitting appointments for the hybrid prosthesis are the same as those described earlier in this chapter. Because of fixture position and intermaxillary space the UCLA-type abutment was used for this patient.

Laboratory

A matrix of the trial setup is made. Gold cylinders with guide pins are placed as previously described. Wax is flowed from an eyedropper into the matrix around the guide pins and gold cylinders. The waxing is carved and refined around the gold cylinders. Buccal and incisal areas are cut back 1.5 mm to 2 mm for porcelain application (Fig. 4-51). A 1 mm finish line is maintained on the palatal slope of the buccal cusps (Fig. 4-52). At least 2 mm of wax is cut back (palatal to the finish line) for light-cured resin application. Plastic retentive beads and undercuts are placed for composite retention. Investing, casting, and reclaiming are accomplished as described in Chapter 3.

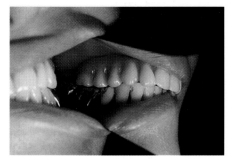

Fig. 4-37

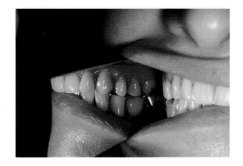

Fig. 4-38

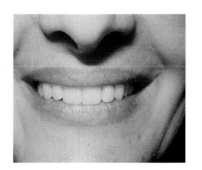

Fig. 4-39

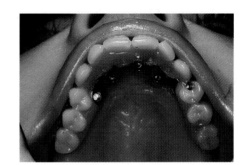

Fig. 4-40

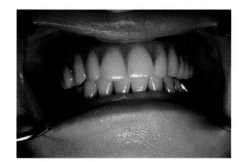

Fig. 4-41

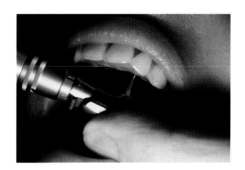

Fig. 4-42

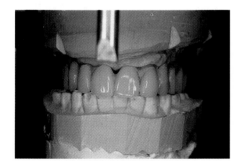

Fig. 4-43

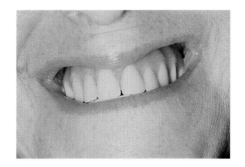

Fig. 4-44

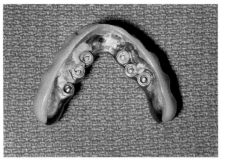

Fig. 4-45

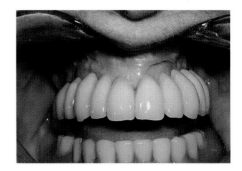

Fig. 4-46

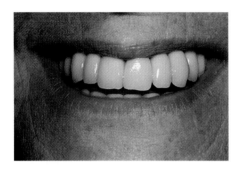

Fig. 4-47

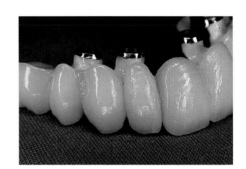

Fig. 4-48

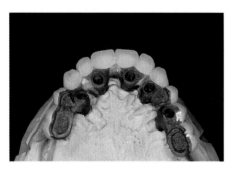

Fig. 4-49

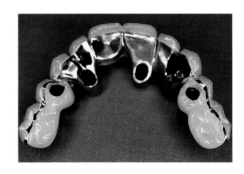

Fig. 4-50

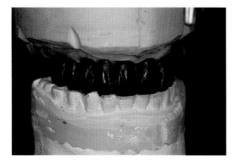

Fig. 4-51

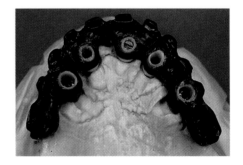

Fig. 4-52

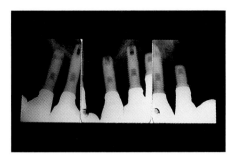

Fig. 4-53

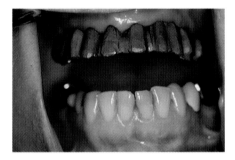

Fig. 4-54

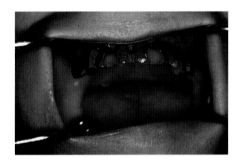

Fig. 4-55

Clinical

The framework is placed on the fixtures and checked for accurate abutment-framework interface. All submucosal fixture framework interfaces, such as UCLA or EsthetiCone abutments, require radiographic verification of fit, since visual inspection is impossible (Fig. 4-53). Inaccurate interface or pain experienced by the patient when the gold abutment screws are tightened requires framework sectioning and solder index (Figs. 4-54 and 4-55).

Laboratory

The metal framework is finished to receive porcelain application. Opaque is applied and fired to the frame (Fig. 4-56). A full porcelain contour is designed, and the first bake is completed (Fig. 4-57). Adjustments are made as necessary, with anatomical contours as designed. Bisque trial fitting is returned for esthetic evaluation and fitting (Fig. 4-58).

Clinical

The transmucosal abutments are removed and the prosthesis is seated. The fixture or abutment-framework interface is checked for accuracy. Lip support, incisal edge position, porcelain contours, and midline are evaluated and modified. The porcelain value, hue, and chroma are evaluated for modification and staining. When the porcelain contours and esthetics have been approved, the prosthesis is ready for posterior composite placement. Centric relation records are made, and the prosthesis is removed. The transmucosal abutments are placed on the fixtures and tightened.

Laboratory

When the bisqued prosthesis is returned, any esthetic corrections are made, and the prosthesis is glazed and polished. Protective measures (as previously documented) should be continually followed, thereby preventing damage of the interface surfaces (Fig. 4-59). The occlusal retentive areas that will receive the composite are metal treated, and microfilled composite is processed to framework. The completed prosthesis is polished and returned to the clinic for delivery to the patient (Fig. 4-60).

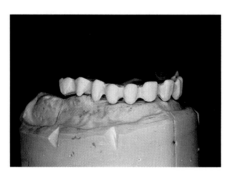

Fig. 4-56

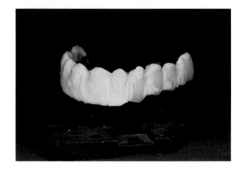

Fig. 4-57

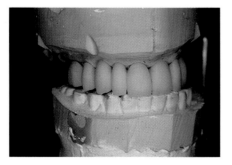

Fig. 4-58

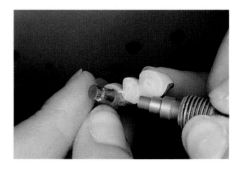

Fig. 4-59

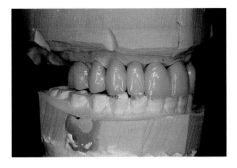

Fig. 4-60

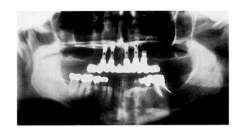

Fig. 4-61

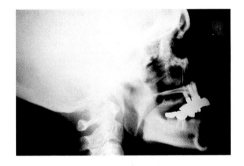

Fig. 4-62

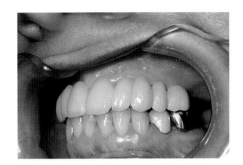

Fig. 4-63

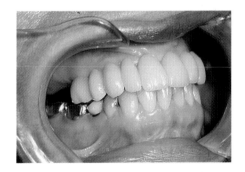

Fig. 4-64

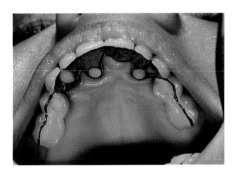

Fig. 4-65

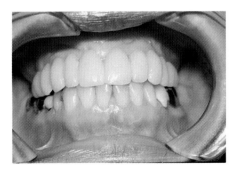

Fig. 4-66

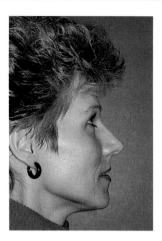

Fig. 4-67

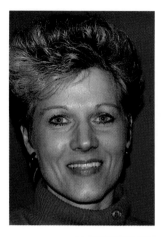

Fig. 4-68

Clinical

The maxillary combination prosthesis is seated. The interfaces are checked for accuracy radiographically. Occlusal ribbon and shimstock are used to perfect the occlusion. A laboratory remount may be used for occlusal adjustment also. After the prosthesis is polished, it is seated, and the gold screws are tightened, using the torque wrench. Temporary fillings are placed in the screw access holes (Figs. 4-61 through 4-68).

5

Tissue-Integrated Single Tooth Prosthesis

Traditional methods of replacing individually missing teeth include removable partial dentures, tooth-supported fixed bridges, and resin-retained bridges, such as the Maryland Bridge. The removable partial denture is the least desirable; however, it is the least expensive restoration. The removable partial denture requires an essential amount of metal framework and tooth support to replace a single tooth. Tooth-supported bridgework can functionally and esthetically replace a missing tooth with excellent long-term results. However, bridge preparation may involve reducing minimally restored or virgin teeth. The abutments are susceptible to recurrent decay. Decay removal may require removing and destroying the bridge, with subsequent cost for a remake. The resin-retained bridge requires minimal tooth preparation; however, short abutments may hinder its retention. Also, the graying of teeth may occur through the translucency of the tooth structure because of the reflection of the bonded metal.

The single tooth implant prosthesis eliminates the drawbacks inherent in a removable partial denture or in resin bridges. Virgin and minimally restored natural teeth are not reduced for abutments, and decay is not a factor. The single tooth implant prosthesis is retrievable for repair or modification, and may be the most cost effective replacement over a period of time. Drawbacks include the initial cost of surgical and prosthetic procedures. If the tooth that is to be replaced is still present, a 6- to 12-month healing time may be necessary after the extraction and before placing the implant. Another 4- to 6-month integration time is necessary before abutment surgery and prosthetic procedures may begin. A treatment partial, or other provisional restoration, must be used in the interim.

Several abutments and techniques are available for single tooth restorations. They have similar or different indications, depending upon the clinical situation.

Indications for single tooth implant-retained prosthesis include tooth loss caused by traumatically avulsed teeth, partial anodontia, cleft palate, and internal or external resorption.

Traumatically avulsed teeth may be repositioned after endodontic treatment and may be crowned if discoloration occurs. Long-term prognosis is unpredictable and an implant prosthesis provides long-term predictability. Patients with congenitally missing teeth and unrestored remaining natural dentition are often ideal candidates for an implant prosthesis. Missing maxillary lateral incisors are found in a small percentage of the population and have often been treated by orthodontically moving cuspids into the lateral incisor position—a solution which effects an esthetic and functional compromise. Orthodontic positioning that is used to provide coronal and apical space for implant placement must be precise. Excellent esthetic results can be achieved with a final implant-retained prosthesis that restores the lateral incisor to its proper size and contour. Cleft palate patients often are missing a lateral incisor. Bone grafting, implant placement, and prosthetic single tooth replacement can effect restoration for these patients with excellent esthetics.

Treatment Planning

Mounted study casts, radiographs, and photographs are necessary for surgical and prosthetic planning. Inadequate space for fixture placement may require orthodontic consultation, as well. Bone quality and quantity, condition and spacing of adjacent natural dentition, intermaxillary space, and soft tissue contours are evaluated. The surgeon determines space and bone quality for fixture placement. Adjacent natural dentition must be caries free, with no periapical pathology. Intermaxillary space may be less than prosthetic component requirements. Orthodontics may be necessary to create adequate intermaxillary space, especially in patients with congenital anodontia. Soft tissue deficits caused by trauma or extraction may require soft tissue management to create ideal gingival contours. Treatment partials provide information on contours and space for the final implant-retained prosthesis and may be used as a guide for fixture placement.

After surgical, orthodontic, and restorative consultations have occurred, fixture placement is completed. Seven to 10 days after surgery the treatment partial, if present, is relined with a tissue treatment material. A definitive reline is completed after healing is complete.

After adequate time for osseointegration has occurred, the abutment surgery is completed. A temporary healing abutment is placed by the surgeon at this time.

Clinical Procedures

Seven to 10 days after abutment surgery an initial alginate impression is made. The treatment partial is tissue treated at this time. *Soft tissues may be swollen, so abutment selection is not made until 2 weeks of additional healing have occurred.*

Abutment Design

Single tooth abutments must be antirotational in design. The fixture-abutment interface must interlock to prevent rotation. The abutment screw must withstand high enough torquing forces to prevent it from becoming loose, yet the force must not be so strong that it will fracture the abutment screw. The Branemark CeraOne abutment was designed with those requirements in mind. It is machined, with a 1 mm to 5 mm collar height to allow a subgingival margin placement and an esthetic emergence profile for the implant prosthesis (Figs. 5-1 and 5-2). The abutment has an internal and external hexagonal design that is retained with a gold alloy screw. This design enables the abutment and fixture to interlock internally, while the external hexagon keeps the implant prosthesis from rotating on the abutment. The gold alloy screw secures the fixture abutment unit and is torqued to 32 Ncm. A countertorque instrument *must* be used for torquing because manual torquing cannot reach the required 32 Ncm. The screw is designed with a square recess that resists stripping with the high torquing forces. The previous titanium screws could only be tightened to 20 Ncm, and abutment loosening was a problem.

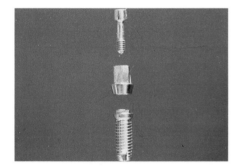

Fig. 5-1

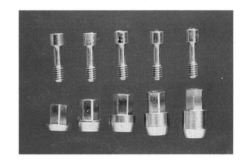

Fig. 5-2

Abutment Selection

Approximately 4 weeks after abutment surgery, tissue healing should be completed, and the abutment collar size is determined. The temporary healing abutment is removed using a slotted or hexagonal screwdriver. Topical anesthetic is introduced, using cotton pellets that are the diameter of the abutment. The pellets prevent tissue collapse until the measurement for collar height can be determined. A periodontal probe is used to measure the distance between the fixture and the gingival surface. After this measurement is recorded, an abutment is selected that has a collar length that is 2 mm to 3 mm less than the distance between the fixture and the gingival surface. The gold screw is placed in the abutment, and the components are seated on the fixture, using the manual countertorque device (Figs. 5-3 and 5-4). The square-headed screwdriver is used to tighten the gold screw (Fig. 5-5). The abutment *must* seat completely on the hexagonal portion of the fixture. As the manual counter-torque device is rotated slightly, the abutment can be felt to slip onto the hexagonal of the fixture. The gold alloy screw is *hand tightened*, and a radiograph is made, aiming the beam parallel to the abutment-fixture interface to verify the seating (Figs. 5-6 and 5-7). While the radiograph is being developed, the blue nylon impression coping is placed on the external hexagonal portion of the abutment to prevent soft tissue collapse.

The nylon impression piece is internally hexagonal to allow a press fit on the hexagonal portion of the abutment (Fig. 5-8). After radiographic verification of the abutment seating, an open window custom tray is tried in the patient's mouth to ensure the path of insertion (Fig. 5-9). Any interferences with the tray placement are eliminated. A medium viscosity polyvinyl siloxane impression material is used to make the impression (Fig. 5-10). After the appropriate adhesive is applied on the tray, the impression material is loaded into the tray; it is also distributed around the impression coping, using a syringe. Hydrostatic pressure and tissue pressure may slightly unseat the coping; therefore, the coping is reseated before placing the impression tray in the patient's mouth. The tray is seated, engaging the impression coping through the tray window. Excess impression material is removed from around the coping, and autopolymerizing resin is used to secure the coping to the impression tray (Fig. 5-11). After the impression has set, it is removed from the mouth (Fig. 5-12). An interocclusal record, a shade selection, and an impression of the opposing arch are made at this time. A temporary crown or the healing abutment is replaced.

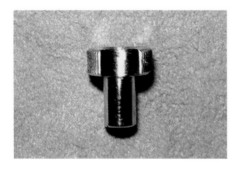

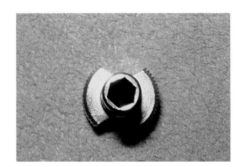

Fig. 5-3   Fig. 5-4

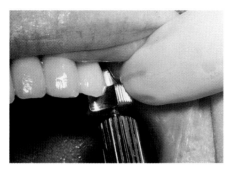

Fig. 5-5

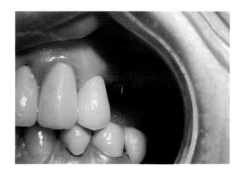

Fig. 5-6

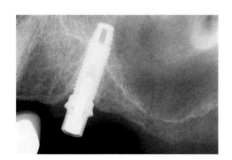

Fig. 5-7

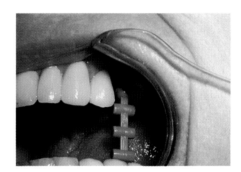

Fig. 5-8

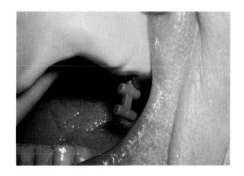

Fig. 5-9

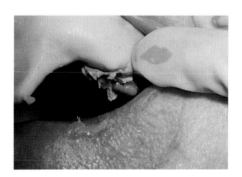

Fig. 5-10

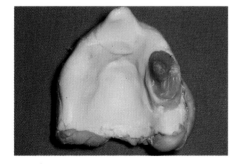

Fig. 5-11

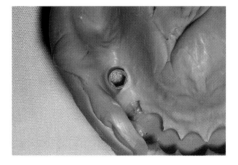

Fig. 5-12

Laboratory Procedures

Pouring the Master Cast

The fixture replica is placed on the inferior surface of the CeraOne impression coping (Figs. 5-13 and 5-14), engaging the internal hex, and held in place by a compression fit of the impression coping. The cast can be poured by using either of the following two methods:

1. Before the master cast is poured, a soft tissue conditioning material can be painted at the gingival area to create a flexible and lifelike margin—an emergence profile (Fig. 5-15).
2. A thin layer of utility wax is placed on the gingival area of the impression coping to inhibit the coping from adhering to the diestone of the cast (Figs. 5-16 and 5-17). This procedure eliminates the possibility of fracturing the master cast upon separation of the impression tray from the cast.

If the second method is used, a special treatment of the master cast is performed to allow fixture interface verification by removing the diestone from the lingual surface of the fixture replica site. Bite relations are verified and the master cast is mounted on a semiadjustable articulator.

Laboratory Procedures

Ceramic caps made from densely sintered aluminum oxide are specially designed for use with the CeraOne abutments (Fig. 5-18 and 5-19). This all-ceramic implant prosthesis offers both optimal esthetics and strength. The cap comes in a short and long length; the cap that is selected should ensure as much support as possible for the finished crown, while it allows for an even layer of porcelain (Figs. 5-20 and 5-21).

The core is manufactured in one shade and can be adjusted by adding an aluminum oxide–core porcelain, such as Vita Dur N HiCeram core material, which is reinforced with 45% to 50% aluminum oxide particles. The porcelain must be well condensed and vacuum fired to eliminate pores in the crystalline ceramic (Fig. 5-22). An all-ceramic crown porcelain, such as Vita Dur N, must be used and can be directly stacked to the core material. The porcelain should be manipulated while wet and not allowed to dry out. Firing should be done slowly to allow any porosities to disappear. The porcelain must not reach the maximum firing temperature before 5 minutes of time has elapsed. Prolonged firing under vacuum at the maximum firing temperature should be avoided, since the glass phase can form bubbles or swell at these temperatures.

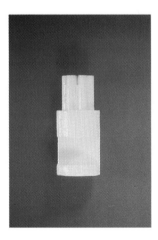

Fig. 5-13

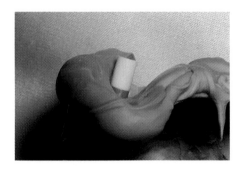

Fig. 5-14

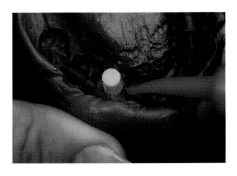

Fig. 5-15

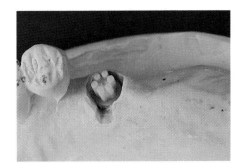

Fig. 5-16

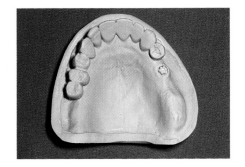

Fig. 5-17

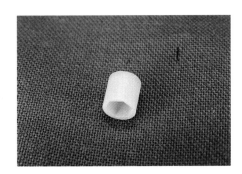

Fig. 5-18

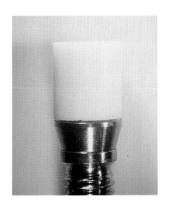

Fig. 5-19

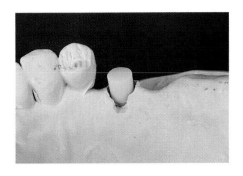

Fig. 5-20

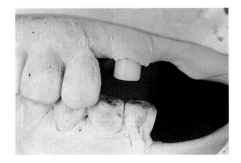

Fig. 5-21

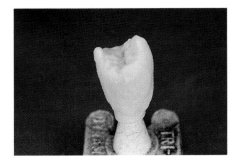

Fig. 5-22

To avoid porcelain with pores, the vacuum must be broken when the aluminum oxide–reinforced porcelain reaches the firing temperature recommended by the manufacturer. After the vacuum has been broken, the aluminum oxide–reinforced porcelain can be safely fired at atmospheric pressure for a long time. If the firing times are too short, the glass phase does not have time to become viscous enough to flow and bond chemically to the aluminum oxide crystals. Tests have shown that complete bonding to the cap can be achieved after 2 minutes.

The cores are adjusted (if necessary) with a diamond bur. The porcelain will bond chemically to the core, so the surface need not be ground to obtain an even porcelain application. The thickness of the core wall should not be less than 0.05 mm on the larger surfaces. For small areas, the cap wall thickness can be slightly less. Before firing takes place, the core should be washed in a solution of diluted hydrofluoric acid for 5 minutes and then carefully cleaned in an ultrasonic bath. As an alternative the core can also be cleaned by means of blasting with pure aluminum oxide powder.

Core material is applied in two firings. This porcelain powder should be mixed with the liquid supplied by the manufacturer. The first layer of porcelain should be thin. Fill all unevenness, wetting the entire surface to minimize the risk for porosities. The porcelain should be fired at 1130° C. The second layer of porcelain is fired at 1120° C, and after this firing the surface should be similar to an eggshell to spread reflected light better.

When the dentin material is fired, work is facilitated by applying a little petroleum jelly to the replica to help keep the crown in place and to minimize the risk of the porcelain attaching itself to the inside of the crown. The firing is done carefully so that the jelly will not get on the outside of the ceramic core. The crown is built up by using the traditional porcelain layering techniques. The crown is glazed after clinical trial fitting has been performed (Figs. 5-23 and 5-24).

Clinical

Bisque Trial Fitting/Delivery

The finished prosthesis is first seated on an extra CeraOne abutment to evaluate the fit. Retention and complete seating are evaluated. Internal debris or flashing may prevent complete seating on the abutment. A disclosing solution is used to show the areas of interference, and these are removed. The healing cap or provisional restoration is removed. If not previously completed on bisque evaluation, the prosthesis is seated, the proximal contacts are checked and adjusted, and a radiograph is made to survey the complete seating. The occlusion is then adjusted to allow light contact; however, *no* contact is allowed in eccentric positions. After the restoration is reglazed and polished (if necessary) it is ready for cementation. The electric torque converter with the square-headed driver is used for final tightening of the gold alloy screw (Figs. 5-25 and 5-26). *The countertorque device must be used to prevent stripping the fixture from the bone.* The countertorque device is first seated on the abutment and checked for lack of rotation. The square-headed driver is used to engage the gold alloy screw (Fig. 5-27). The electric torque converter is set to 32 Ncm at the low setting. The footpedal is then used to completely tighten the screw. A cotton pellet is placed over the gold screw inside the abutment. The choice of cement depends on retention between the abutment and the prosthesis. In many instances, temporary cement will retain the restoration and allow for possible retrieval of the unit if necessary. If retention is not high, a more permanent cement must be used. Only a thin layer of cement is used inside the restoration to prevent subgingival cement, which may be difficult to remove. After cementation and seat verification, hygiene instructions are given to the patient. The single tooth prosthesis is checked according to protocol at follow-up appointments (Figs. 5-28 and 5-29).

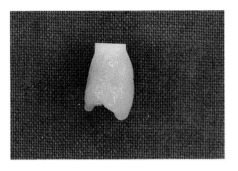

Fig. 5-23

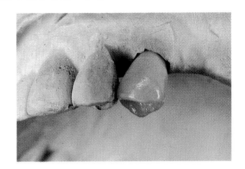

Fig. 5-24

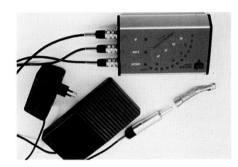

Fig. 5-25

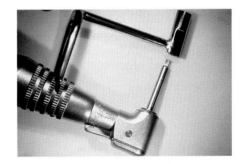

Fig. 5-26

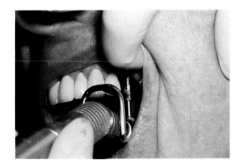

Fig. 5-27

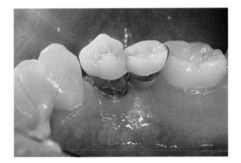

Fig. 5-28

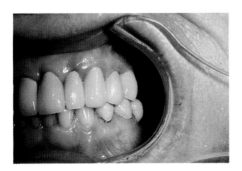

Fig. 5-29

CeraOne Metal Coping

Laboratory Waxing Procedure

When the CeraOne is waxed with a metal coping, the design and fabrication of the substructure must be considered. A plastic burnout replica pattern is available for casting a CeraOne metal coping.

The burnout replica pattern is placed on the plastic abutment replica, the casts are closed in centric relationship, and the intermaxillary space is adjusted for the metal and porcelain additions. The burnout replica is shortened to allow adequate porcelain thickness. The area around the abutment replica and burnout replica is lubricated on the master cast to facilitate easy removal between it and the waxed pattern. Inlay wax is applied to the burnout replica, and a wax contour of the prosthesis is fabricated. The esthetic, hygiene, and tissue emergence profiles are established. The wax pattern is cut back for proper thickness of porcelain application (Figs. 5-30 and 5-31). The facial ceramic metal junction can be carried subgingivally to aid in the emergence profile (Fig. 5-32). The wax pattern is indirectly sprued (Fig. 5-33) with an 8 gauge sprue at the lingual surface and removed from the plastic abutment replica.

Phosphate investment with proper expansion is recommended to ensure a precise fit between the fabricated casting and the CeraOne abutment replica. A manufacturer's investment procedure is recommended. An alloy is selected with a tensile strength in the area of 150,000. (Alloys designed for ceramic application have a greater tensile strength, thus their selection for prostheses when porcelain is to be applied is recommended.) An extra CeraOne abutment should be used to verify fit and interface during the reclaiming and metal finishing of the cast coping. The finished coping now can be returned to the clinic for the metal trial and for the interoral fit evaluation, or porcelain procedures may begin. The cast coping is prepared, and the traditional opaque and porcelain techniques are performed (Fig. 5-34). After the porcelain procedures are completed, the prosthesis is returned to the clinic for bisque trial fitting (Fig. 5-35).

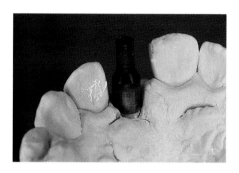

Fig. 5-30

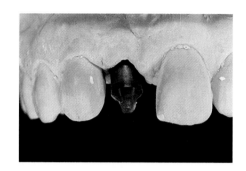

Fig. 5-31

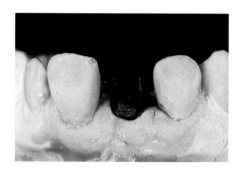

Fig. 5-32

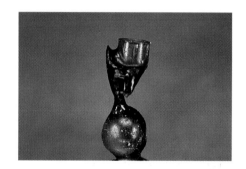

Fig. 5-33

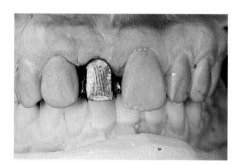

Fig. 5-34

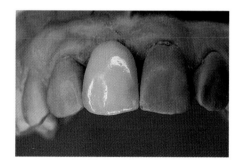

Fig. 5-35

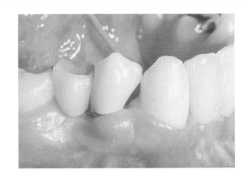

Fig. 5-36

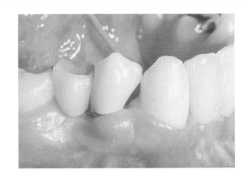

Fig. 5-37

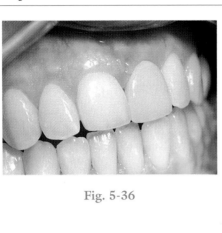

Fig. 5-38

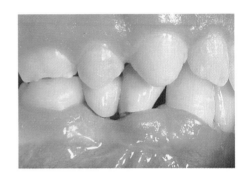

Fig. 5-39

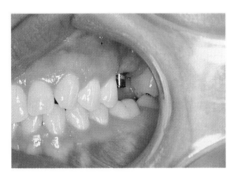

Fig. 5-40

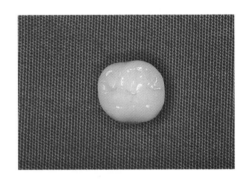

Fig. 5-41

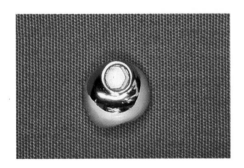

Fig. 5-42

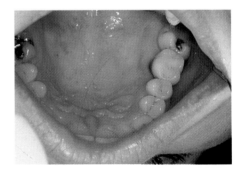

Fig. 5-43

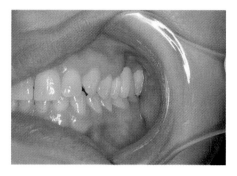

Fig. 5-44

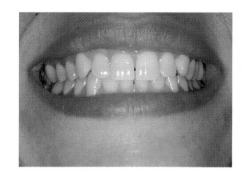

Fig. 5-45

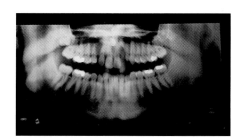

Fig. 5-46

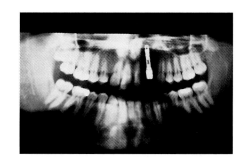

Fig. 5-47

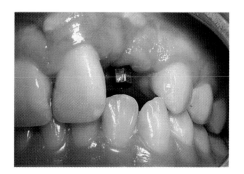

Fig. 5-48

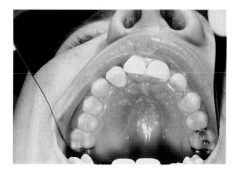

Fig. 5-49

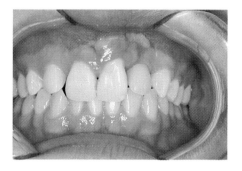

Fig. 5-50

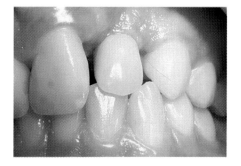

Fig. 5-51

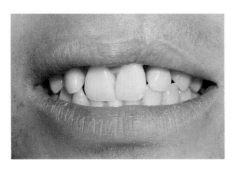

Fig. 5-52

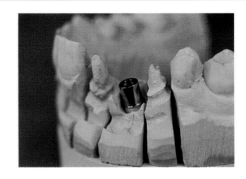

Fig. 5-53

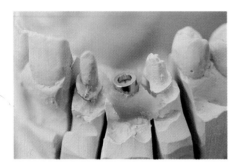

Fig. 5-54

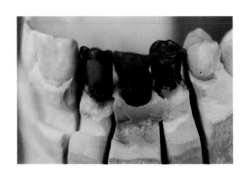

Fig. 5-55

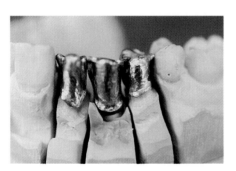

Fig. 5-56

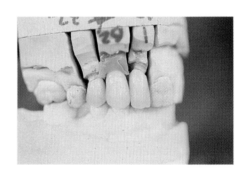

Fig. 5-57

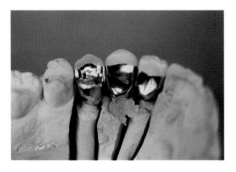

Fig. 5-58

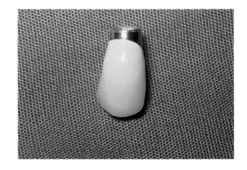

Fig. 5-59

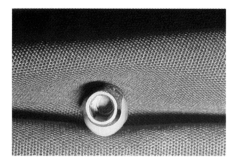

Fig. 5-60

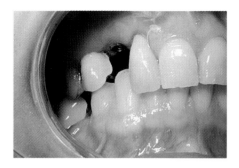

Fig. 5-61

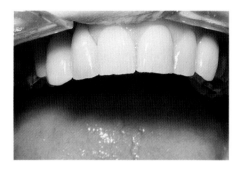

Fig. 5-62

Clinical Delivery

Clinical procedures for the CeraOne metal coping have been discussed previously (the ceramic cap procedure). Again, the implant prosthesis should be light in occlusion to deter the possibility of a load-carrying compromise of the fixture. A metal trial fitting is not necessary with the CeraOne; however, an alternative is a bisque trial fitting; both the casting fit and the esthetic evaluation can be accomplished at the same time, and the contacts can be adjusted with the adjacent teeth. Radiographic verification should be performed to ensure that the casting is seated onto the abutment and that the interface between the cast coping and the abutment is closed. If the occlusion requires adjustment, it is accomplished after verification of seating. Preferably, light contact is established in centric occlusion and functional contact is avoided. Occlusal adjustment should be made to prevent the implant prosthesis from taking the whole load in any position (Fig. 5-36).

The crown is returned to the laboratory for final staining, glazing, and polishing, before returning it to the clinic for seating. A metal-supported ceramic prosthesis is recommended for all posterior single tooth restorations. Figs. 5-37 through 5-39 demonstrate a ceramic metal prosthesis for congenital anodontia. Figs. 5-40 through 5-45 show single molar replacement in the maxillary posterior. The patient shown in Figs. 5-46 through 5-52 had a bone graft to repair a cleft palate defect. After the grafting procedure had been performed, fixture placement and single tooth replacement were done. Figs. 5-53 through 5-62 illustrate fabrication and replacement of tooth #6, using a machined gold cylinder and porcelain application, along with conventional porcelain to metal restorations on teeth #5 and #7.

CHAPTER

6

Partially Edentulous Fixed-Implant Prosthesis

Partial edentulism has traditionally been treated with removable partial dentures when the natural dentition is insufficient to support the conventional fixed prosthesis. Removable partial dentures include potential for tissue irritation because of prosthesis movement, nonphysiological forces generated on tooth abutments, esthetics compromise caused by retentive elements, and psychological adjustment to wearing a removable prosthesis. The fixed implant-retained prosthesis (FIRP) compensates for the disadvantages of a removable partial denture by eliminating prosthesis movement, dependency on natural dentition for retention, and the stigma of a removable prosthesis.

Tooth-supported, fixed partial dentures also provide functional and esthetic replacements for missing teeth. Abutments require reduction and preparation before prosthesis fabrication. Multiple unrestored teeth may be necessary as abutments for a long span fixed prosthesis. These abutments are susceptible to decay and periodontal disease. The FIRP spares virgin teeth from preparation and is not susceptible to decay. FIRPs are retrievable by design for repair and modification. The initial cost of an FIRP may be higher than for a tooth-supported prosthesis, when combining surgical and prosthetic fees. However, the long-term cost may be less because fewer units are involved, an FIRP is retrievable, and it does not decay. Implant loss and component breakage are possible complications with a implant-retained prosthesis.

Treatment Planning

Parameters affecting treatment planning include adequate bone for implant placement, position of available bone, intermaxillary space, smile line, patient expectations, and finances.

An intraoral exam is completed, including the charting of missing teeth, existing restorations, and caries; also, radiographs are made. Alginate impressions of both dental arches are made, along with interocclusal records. The mounted diagnostic casts and radiographs are used when the surgeon and the restorative dentist consult. The casts are also used for fabrication of surgical stents by the dental technician (see Chapter 2).

After surgical and prosthetic consultation, the surgeon, the restorative dentist, and the dental technician consider a treatment plan (discussed in Chapter 1). Mounted casts, radiographs, and pictures showing facial profile, full face, and smile line are used to determine the number and position of implants to produce a functional and esthetic result. A tooth-supported surgical stent is fabricated as a guide for implant placement during surgery.

Clinical

After the fixture is placed, a healing time of 7 to 10 days is necessary without a prosthesis being worn. The existing definitive or treatment partial is relieved and relined with a tissue conditioning material. This lining is replaced as needed until healing is complete. A more definitive reline is completed at this time. The patient is advised to return to the clinic for prosthesis adjustment at the first sign of soreness or irritation.

The abutment operation is completed at the proper time, followed by 7 to 10 days without a prosthesis. The prosthesis is relieved, allowing excess clearance so that no acrylic resin or metal touches the abutments, and a soft reline with tissue conditioner is completed. Preliminary impressions are made with an alginate or hydrocolloid impression material. Interocclusal records are made at this time, also.

Laboratory

Laboratory abutment replicas are placed in the impression before pouring in the diestone. The replicas are necessary for determining exact fixture angulation for abutment selection. At this time the mounted casts are used with guide pins in the replicas for diagnostic waxing. Fixture position, angulation, intermaxillary space, smile line, patient expectations, and opposing arch help determine which abutment will be used in the final restoration. Abutment choice will determine the impression technique. Abutment options include the traditional abutment, angulated abutment, EsthetiCone abutment, and the UCLA abutment.

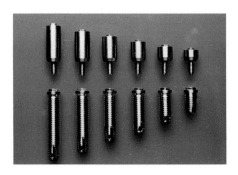

Fig. 6-1

Traditional Abutment

This is the abutment of choice in clinical situations when adequate intermaxillary space and ideal implant position and angulation are present (Fig. 6-1). Esthetics must not be compromised by abutment and gold cylinder metal display. Common areas of use are maxillary and mandibular posterior bridges and mandibular anterior areas. The patient is involved in abutment selection to avoid dissatisfaction with metal display. If the patient shows abutment metal when smiling or talking and finds this objectionable, then an alternative abutment is chosen. The following are several advantages to the traditional abutment:

1. Titanium interface
2. Hygiene access
3. Machined interface visible supragingivally
4. Longest clinical trials
5. Gold screw failsafe

This abutment is made of surgical grade titanium that is identical to the implant. The interface is of similar metals, which eliminates the possibility of a galvanic reaction. Prosthetic design usually involves a hygienic pontic and open embrasures for access for cleaning. The abutment is machined rather than cast, which allows maximum interface accuracy. The interface between the prosthetic framework and the transmucosal abutment can be visualized when checking for passive fit. The passive and intimate fit is mandatory to minimize torquing fixtures when tightening the framework. Ill-fitting framework can be a cause of loss of osseointegration and fixture loss. Components, such as gold screws and abutment screws, are subject to fracture with ill-fitting frameworks. The traditional abutment was used in most reports on long-term implant success. New abutments do not have the long-term trials by which to judge success.

Clinical Procedures

Diagnostic casts made previously are used to make custom trays (Figs. 6-2 through 6-5). The open window design is used as previously documented in Chapter 3. The titanium hemostats and hex wrench are used to assure abutment screw tightness. All calculus and plaque are removed from the abutments. Impression copings are placed and visualized for intimate interface with abutments circumferentially (Figs. 6-7 and 6-8).

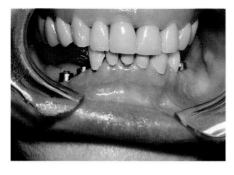

Fig. 6-2

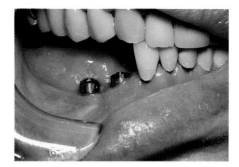

Fig. 6-3

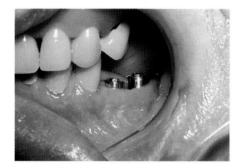

Fig. 6-4

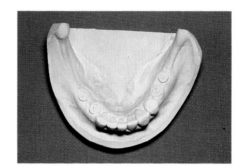

Fig. 6-5

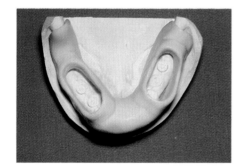

Fig. 6-6

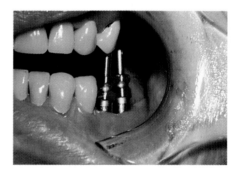

Fig. 6-7

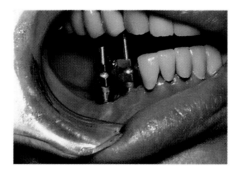

Fig. 6-8

Long guide pins are used when space allows. Short guide pins may be necessary in the posterior region. If fixtures are placed too close together or if they are placed at an angle that will not allow the square impression coping to be used, tapered impression copings may be used alternatively. It should be noted that air may be introduced into the master cast because of the removal and replacement of the tapered impression copings into the impression. The impression tray is tried in the mouth and excess tray material is trimmed to allow ease of insertion (Fig. 6-9). Wax is sealed over the window, and the tray is placed in the mouth to record guide pin and coping position (Fig. 6-10). Adhesive is applied to the tray. A medium viscosity vinyl polysiloxane impression material is mixed and placed in the tray. A crown and bridge syringe is used to inject impression material around the impression coping and the tray is seated. Guide pins are exposed, and the tray is removed (Fig. 6-11).

The impression is prepared and poured in the stone as described previously (Figs. 6-12 and 6-13).

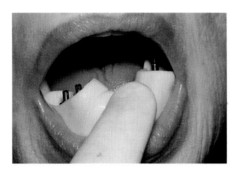

Fig. 6-9

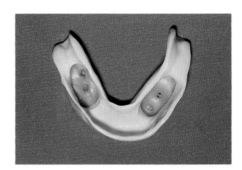

Fig. 6-10

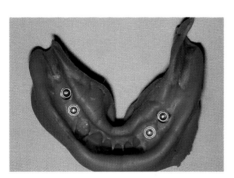

Fig. 6-11

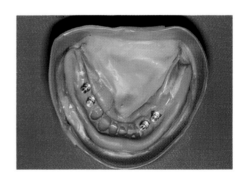

Fig. 6-12

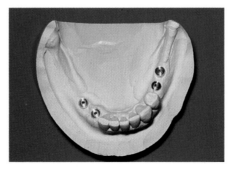

Fig. 6-13

Interoral Bite Registration

If the final prosthesis in an implant system is retained interorally with set screws, the interocclusal records can be fabricated and stabilized by screw components during the bite registration procedures.

On each side, two impression copings (that have been cut in half) are placed on the brass abutment replicas and secured in place with guide pin screws (Fig. 6-14). The ridge area around the brass replicas (and distally) is blocked out, and a trough is formed with utility wax to receive self-polymerizing acrylic (Fig. 6-15). The trough is filled with the acrylic to the top edge of the impression coping and placed in a pressure-curing pot for processing. After the wax has cured, the utility wax is removed from the tray, the excess acrylic is trimmed away, and the inferior surfaces are contoured (Fig. 6-16). Bite registration wax is applied to the occlusal surface and returned to the clinic for bite registration procedures (Figs. 6-17 and 6-18).

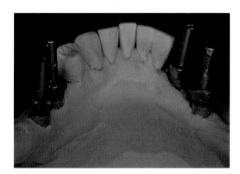

Fig. 6-14

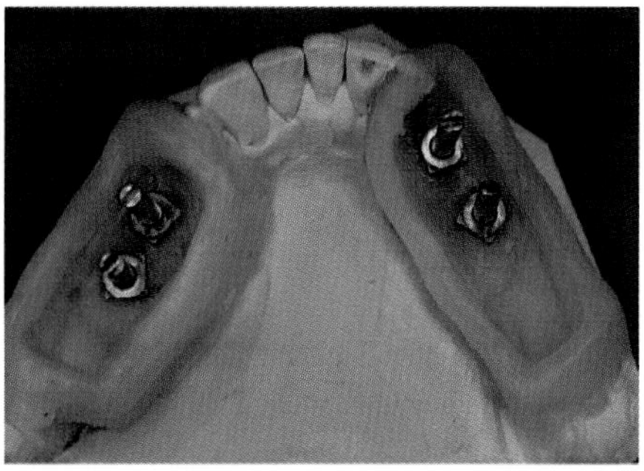

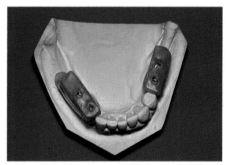

Fig. 6-15

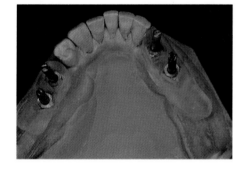

Fig. 6-16

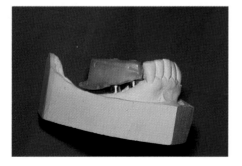

Fig. 6-17

Fig. 6-18

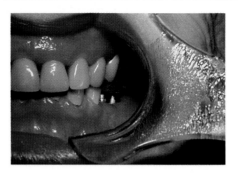

Fig. 6-19

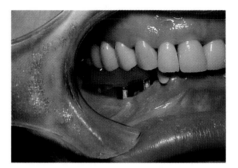

Fig. 6-20

When the usual preparatory clinical procedures are completed, the occlusion rims are inserted and secured with short guide pins (Figs. 6-19 and 6-20). The occlusal rim material is softened, and the patient is guided into centric relation. The interocclusal records are removed, chilled in cool water, replaced onto the master cast, and returned to the laboratory for cast remount and framework fabrication.

Framework Fabrication

The master cast and opposing arch are mounted on a semiadjustable articulator, and the casts are prepared for framework fabrication (Fig. 6-21). A gold cylinder is placed on each of the brass replicas and is secured with a guide pin. The guide pin screw has been reduced in height and has been reslotted to accommodate the centric occlusal relationship (Fig. 6-22). A full-contour wax pattern is designed with considerations of function and esthetics (Figs. 6-23 and 6-24). A line is scribed on the wax pattern on the lingual surface, halfway between the occlusal surface and the inferior boarder of the wax pattern. On the buccal surface, a 2 mm finishing line is placed around each gold cylinder and the pontic areas. A wax bur is used to reduce the bulk of the wax pattern for allowance of proper thickness of a composite application to the framework. Consideration must be made for mechanical retention of the tooth shade veneering material. Three types of retention used are undercuts, plastic beads, and silicoating (Figs. 6-25 and 6-26).

The wax pattern is indirectly sprued, weighed to determine the amount of required alloy, placed on a sprue former, and invested. The pattern is cast, reclaimed, and placed on the master cast for fit evaluation (Figs. 6-27 and 6-28). The framework is returned to the clinic for an oral fit evaluation.

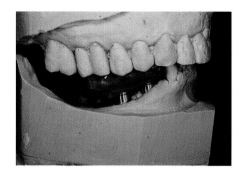

Fig. 6-21

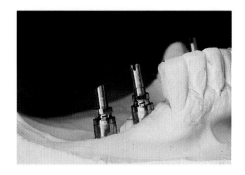

Fig. 6-22

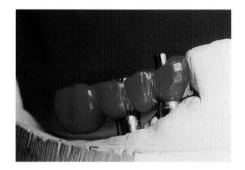

Fig. 6-23

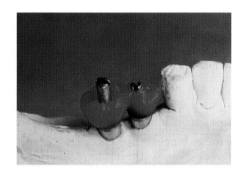

Fig. 6-24

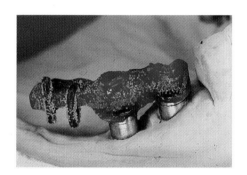

Fig. 6-25

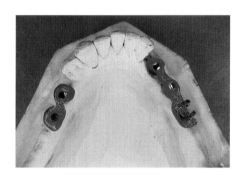

Fig. 6-26

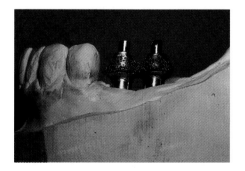

Fig. 6-27

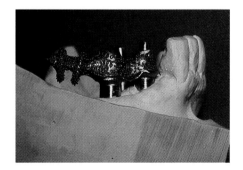

Fig. 6-28

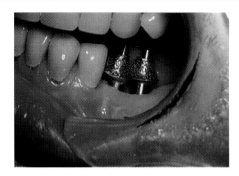
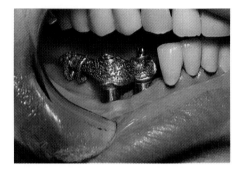

Fig. 6-29   Fig. 6-30

Framework Try-in

The framework is seated passively (Figs. 6-29 and 6-30). If proximal contacts are in metal, they may interfere with complete seating. Disclosing solution is used to identify and to adjust the contacts. The interface between the abutments and the framework is visualized circumferentially. An unacceptable interface is corrected by sectioning and making a solder index (as previously documented). The frame is removed and returned to the laboratory.

Composite Application

When the framework is returned to the laboratory, it is prepared, cleaned, and silicoated, or a bonding agent is applied for the light-cured composite application. The shade of material is selected; the framework is masked with opaque; and the composite is stacked, contoured, and light-cured. Final composite occlusal adjustments and contouring are performed, and the composite is polished (Fig. 6-31). The metal framework is highshined, and the prosthesis is replaced on the master cast for final quality evaluation and inspection.

Clinical Delivery

The prosthesis is again trial fitted, and the interface is verified (Figs. 6-32 and 6-33). Proximal contacts are refined. If the interface is accurate, restorative veneering and interproximal contacts are adjusted, and the abutment screw is checked for tightness. Plaque and calculus are eliminated from the abutment. If the interface is still incorrect, the frame is sectioned, individual interfaces are verified, and a solder index is made. If the interface is correct, the proximal contacts are finished. The occlusion is adjusted, using shimstock as the final check and verifying occlusal contact on the implant prosthesis and adjacent teeth. After the prosthesis is polished, the gold screws are tightened, using the torque wrench. The temporary restorations are placed in the screw access holes. The patient then is instructed by the hygienist in homecare techniques.

Partially Edentulous—EsthetiCone Abutment

The EsthetiCone abutment is designed to be used in multiple fixture situations if the traditional abutment might cause esthetic compromise with the metal display. It is designed to allow esthetic veneering material to be placed subgingivally, thereby avoiding metal display (Figs. 6-34 and 6-35). The abutment is made of surgical grade titanium and is available with 1 mm, 2 mm, and 3 mm collars (Fig. 6-36). The depth of the fixture determines the size of the abutment that must be used. A gold alloy cylinder and a gold screw are used in the fabrication of the metal frameworks—much the same techniques as described in previous chapters (Fig. 6-37).

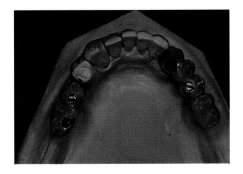

Fig. 6-31

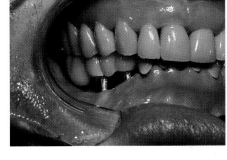

Fig. 6-32

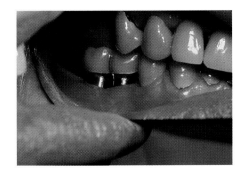

Fig. 6-33

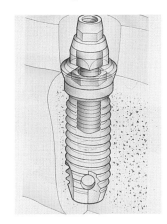

Fig. 6-34

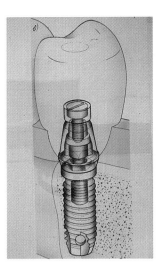

Fig. 6-35

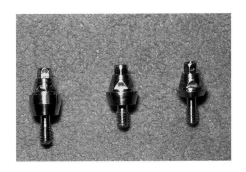

Fig. 6-36

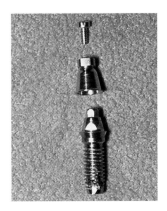

Fig. 6-37

Clinical Procedures

The patient is seen by the clinician 7 to 10 days following abutment surgery. Alginate impressions, as well as an interocclusal registration, are made of the maxilla and mandible. The mounted diagnostic casts are used to determine which type of abutment will be used and for fabricating the custom tray. Determination of abutment collar size should not be made until tissue shrinkage following second stage surgery is complete. At this time the temporary healing abutments are removed, and a periodontal probe is used to measure the distance between the fixture and the gingival surface. Abutments are selected individually for each fixture to allow 2 mm of veneering material to be placed subgingivally. Therefore, the collar on the abutment needs to be at least 2 mm below tissue (Figs. 6-38 through 6-40). The abutment is placed in the manual countertorque device and guided to engage the head of the fixture. A light, back and forth rotation is used to engage the hexagonal portion of the fixture (Fig. 6-41). The hexagonal screwdriver is used to tighten the abutment screw (Fig. 6-42). Radiographs are made of the abutments at this time to ensure complete seating. After seating verification, the mechanical or electric torque drivers are used to tighten the abutment screws to 20 Ncm.

Two types of impression copings are available: a square type and a cylindrical type (Figs. 6-42 and 6-43). The square impression is preferred. The impression copings are screwed into place on the abutments, using guide pins (Fig. 6-44). An open-window custom tray is placed in the mouth to check for guide pin and coping clearance (Fig. 6-45). After the wax window is placed and the guide pin imprints are captured in wax (as previously described), adhesive is placed, a polyvinyl siloxane or other impression material is mixed, and the impression is made in the usual manner (Fig. 6-46). After the impression material has set, the guide pins are unscrewed until a clicking sound is heard or felt, and the impression is removed. The plastic healing caps are placed on each abutment to prevent tissue collapse (Fig. 6-47). If an interim prosthesis is present, it is relieved and relined with a tissue conditioning material in the area of the healing caps. An interocclusal record is made at this time.

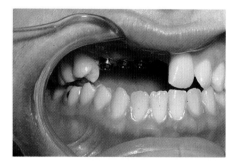

Fig. 6-38

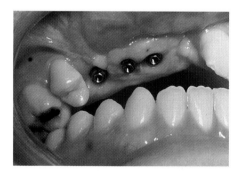

Fig. 6-39

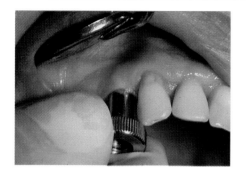

Fig. 6-40

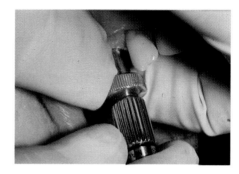

Fig. 6-41

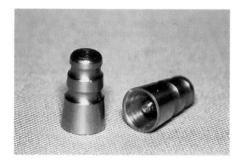

Fig. 6-42

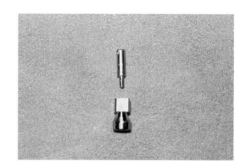

Fig. 6-43

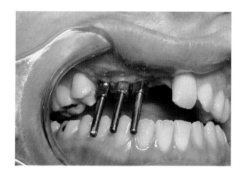

Fig. 6-44

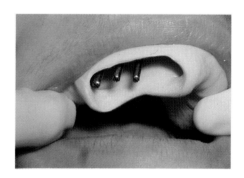

Fig. 6-45

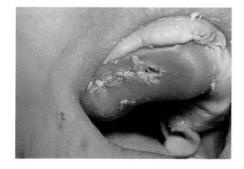

Fig. 6-46

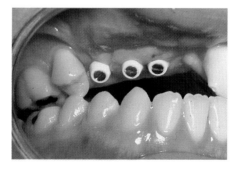

Fig. 6-47

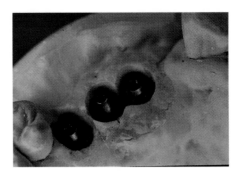

Fig. 6-48

Laboratory Procedures

A cast of the impression can be handled in one of two ways: (1) a small amount of utility wax can be applied around the subgingival area of the impression coping so that the master cast will not fracture upon separation; or (2) tissue conditioner can be painted around the impression coping to simulate the free gingival margin around the abutment (Fig. 6-48). If option 1 is used, the diestone on the lingual side of the abutment is removed to provide access to verify gold cylinder interface seating. Abutment replicas are affixed to the impression coping and secured with guide pins. The impression is cast in diestone, separated and mounted on a semiadjustable articulator.

Waxing Procedures

Tapered gold cylinders are placed on the replicas (Fig. 6-49). The casts are closed into centric relation, and the intermaxillary space is measured. A minimum of 6.7 mm is required between the fixture flange and the opposing dentition for Estheti-Cone components.

Conventional waxing procedures are performed with consideration for type of veneering material that will be used. Design may include metal, porcelain, or microfilled composite, depending on the restorative dentist's preference. The wax pattern is sprued, invested, cast, reclaimed, and returned to the clinic for metal try-in (Figs. 6-50 through 6-56).

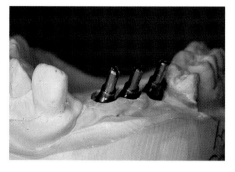

Fig. 6-49

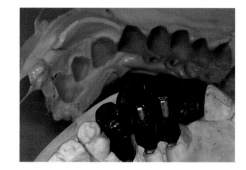

Fig. 6-50

Fig. 6-51

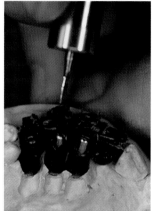

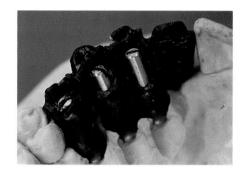

Fig. 6-52

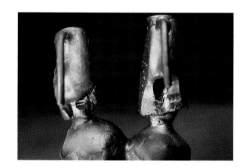

Fig. 6-53

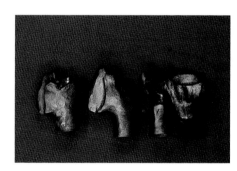

Fig. 6-54

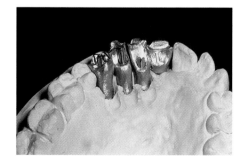

Fig. 6-55

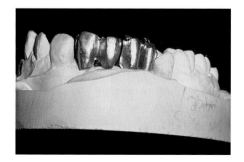

Fig. 6-56

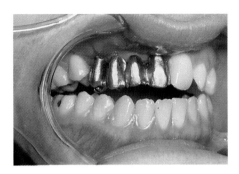

Fig. 6-57

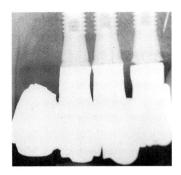

Fig. 6-58

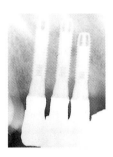

Fig. 6-59

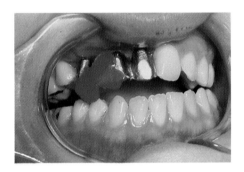

Fig. 6-60

The metal castings are tried in individual units per abutment. One disadvantage with the subgingival margins that exist between the EsthetiCone abutment and prosthetic framework is that the interface accuracy cannot be visualized. Radiograph verification gives a two-dimensional view of the interface, which is affected by radiographic angulation and cannot be verified with complete confidence. Therefore the castings are tried in as individual units (Fig. 6-57). Radiographs are made to evaluate the seating of individual units. Fig. 6-58 shows an example of a distal unit that was incompletely seated because of proximal contact with the adjacent natural tooth. Fig. 6-59 displays radiographic confirmation of the seating after adjustment. Autopolymerizing resin is used for solder indexing, and the castings are removed from the mouth (Fig. 6-60).

Laboratory

Brass replicas are secured to the casting and held in place with guide pins. Undercuts are blocked out with utility wax, and a soldering matrix is constructed from diestone. The casting is placed in a soldering investment, and the soldering is completed (Fig. 6-61); the casting is returned to clinic for a trial fitting.

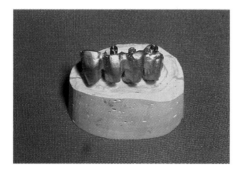

Fig. 6-61

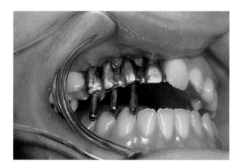

Fig. 6-62

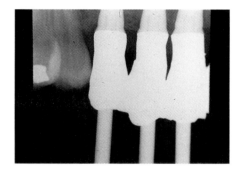

Fig. 6-63

Clinical

The healing caps are removed, and the abutments are cleaned of all debris. The hexagonal wrench is used to verify the abutment tightness. The framework is passively tightened on the abutments (Fig. 6-62). The patient is asked if any pain exists as the screws are tightened. If pain exists, the patient is requested to differentiate between bony fixture pain and soft tissue pain. Often the soft tissues may collapse onto the abutment after the healing caps are removed, and the pinching of tissue during framework seating may be painful. Repeated fixture pain during the process of tightening and loosening screws indicates that torque is being transmitted into the fixtures from an ill-fitting frame, or it may indicate that a fixture has not integrated. Radiographs are made to examine abutment framework interface (Fig. 6-63). Pain or radiographic evidence of poor fit requires framework sectioning and solder indexing, as previously described. If there is a perfect framework fit, it is ready for veneer application.

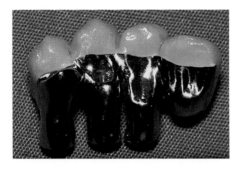

Fig. 6-64

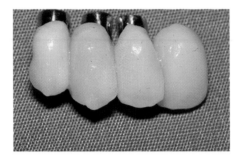

Fig. 6-65

Laboratory

The casting is prepared for opaque and porcelain application. Porcelain is applied by conventional methods: contoured, stained, and glazed. The casting is returned to the clinic for seating (Figs. 6-64 and 6-65).

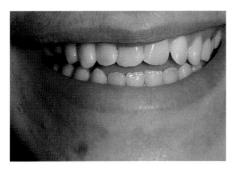

Fig. 6-66

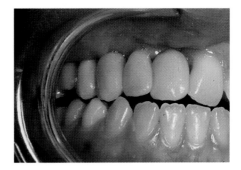

Fig. 6-67

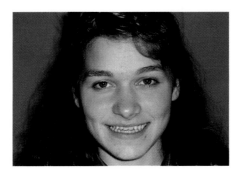

Fig. 6-68

Clinical Delivery

Porcelain application may distort the framework; thus it must be evaluated for fit after porcelain contouring and subsequent porcelain firings. At the delivery appointment, proximal contacts and occlusion are adjusted. The prosthesis is seated and a radiographic evaluation of fit is completed. The prosthesis is seated onto the abutments and one of the torque drivers is used to tighten the gold screws to 10 N/cm (Figs. 6-66 through 6-68). Temporary restoration material is placed in the screw access holes, and oral hygiene instructions are given to the patient.

◆ PARTIALLY EDENTULOUS—UCLA ABUTMENT

This abutment was originally developed to compensate for space and esthetic limitations that are found with the traditional transmucosal abutment. Combined height of the transmucosal abutment and the gold cylinder left no room for restorative material in certain clinical situations.

Display of the transmucosal abutments in esthetic areas is unacceptable in some clinical situations. The UCLA-type abutment is designed to bypass the transmucosal abutment and fit directly on the fixture (Fig. 6-69). This allows for fabrication of a prosthesis in areas where the intermaxillary space precludes the traditional system. Veneering material can also be placed subgingivally, thereby eliminating metal display.

The interface between the implant and abutment is no longer titanium to titanium. Palladium-silver or palladium-gold alloys are most often used in the prosthetic framework. Dissimilar metals in contact may produce a galvanic response. This potential galvanic response is located at the implant-framework interface, which is close to the fixture-bone interface. The UCLA-type abutment in its original form was a plastic sleeve that was used as a matrix for waxing and casting the prosthetic framework. A lapping tool with milling paste is used to refine the framework portion of the framework-fixture interface. This is not a controlled machined surface and because it is located subgingivally, it cannot be verified visually. Castings are individual per implant and are indexed in the mouth for soldering.

A lack of intermaxillary space and a metal display with traditional abutment are indications that it might be wise to consider the use of the UCLA-type abutment (Fig. 6-70).

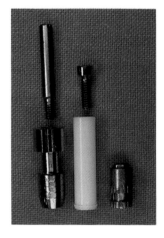

Fig. 6-69

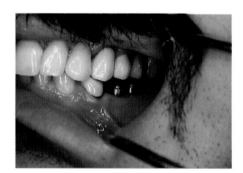

Fig. 6-70

Primary Impressions

The finished prosthesis bypasses the traditional abutment and fits directly on the fixture. The abutment is removed with the hexagonal wrench (Figs. 6-71 and 6-72). Topical anesthetic is placed subgingivally with a cotton pellet. The pellet is large enough to maintain the diameter of the fixture access, and does not allow tissue to collapse. The cotton pellet is removed after 1 minute, and the single tooth impression coping is placed on the fixture; however, the clinician must make sure that the hexagonal head of the wrench is engaged. The guide pin is tightened. An impression tray (as previously described) is adapted, and the impression is made. After the guide pins are loosened, the impression is removed, and cotton pellets with topical anesthetic are applied. The transmucosal abutments then are replaced. An alginate impression of the opposing arch is made, along with an interocclusal record and a facebow transfer.

Laboratory Procedures

Pouring the Impressions

The fixture replicas are placed on the single-tooth impression coping. The subgingival surface of the single tooth impression coping should be covered with a light coat of utility wax so that the master cast will not be fractured when it is separated from the impression tray. The master cast is poured in diestone, using the usual procedures. Interocclusal records are used to mount the master casts on a semiadjustable articulator. The master cast is prepared by removing the lingual stone at the fixture site, exposing the fixture replica. This is done to verify the interface of the UCLA cylinder.

Prostheses are waxed to full contour, allowing access for hygiene. Normal cutback procedures are performed. The interface of the UCLA cylinder will be milled with a lapping procedure after casting. Because of the tolerance changes during the lapping procedures it is not possible to cast two cylinders in a one-piece casting. Therefore, each fixture-framework unit is cast in separate pieces, and a soldering relationship is made in the mouth. The separated wax patterns are individually sprued, invested, cast, reclaimed, and replaced on the master cast for fit verification. The castings are sent to clinic for interoral fit evaluation.

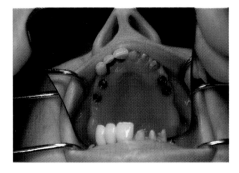

Fig. 6-71

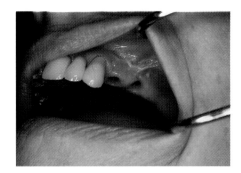

Fig. 6-72

Clinical Framework Trial Fitting and Soldering Index

Individual castings are tried intraorally to verifiy accuracy of fit and to establish a solder matrix. The transmucosal abutments are removed, topical anesthetic is applied, and individual castings are seated. Adjacent castings are aligned, using cuts at the prospective solder joints. Radiographs are made perpendicular to the framework interface to verify the seating. After the seating is verified, a solder index is made using autopolymerizing resin. The framework is removed, the transmucosal abutments are replaced, and the indexed frames are returned to the laboratory for soldering.

Soldering Procedures

Fixture replicas are placed onto the UCLA framework. A soldering index is cast in diestone. The framework is removed and the self-polymerizing resin is burned off. The individual sections are placed onto the soldering index and luted together. The luted framework is removed from the index and invested in a high-heat soldering investment. Soldering procedures are performed and the castings are returned to the clinic for try-in.

Clinical—Soldered Framework Trial Fitting

Usual preliminary procedures are performed. Frameworks are seated and the titanium screws are sequentially tightened. Radiographic verification is completed. The patient is questioned concerning pain around the implants during and after tightening. Soft tissue discomfort is differentiated from bone discomfort. If interface discrepancy is seen on radiographs or if the patient reports bone pain during or after tightening, the framework is sectioned in the appropriate places, and a new solder index is made.

Laboratory Procedures

Fixture replicas are placed onto the framework and held in place with guide pins. The frameworks are replaced into the impression and secured with sticky wax. The subgingival areas are blocked out to the fixture replica interface. The impression is poured in diestone and separated; bite relations are reset and remounted on a semiadjustable articulator.

A combination of buccal porcelain and occlusal light cured resin is used as described in Chapter 4 (Fig. 6-73). The contouring, polishing, and finishing procedures are performed, and the framework is returned to the clinic for insertion (Figs. 6-74 and 6-75).

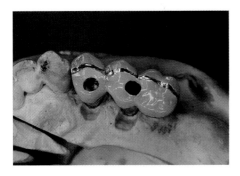

Fig. 6-73

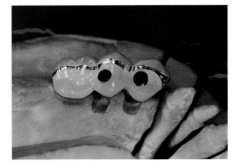

Fig. 6-74

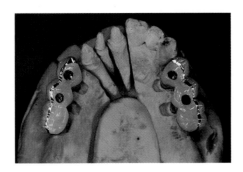

Fig. 6-75

Clinical Seating and Delivery

Abutments are again removed and topical anesthetic is applied. The framework is seated. Proximal contacts are adjusted, using disclosing solution. Radiographic verification of seating is accomplished (Figs. 6-76 and 6-77), followed by occlusal adjustment, until the implant framework and adjacent natural teeth hold shimstock (Figs. 6-78 through 6-83). The prosthesis is polished, and screw access holes are temporarily filled. The patient is seen the following day by the hygienist for complete instructions in hygiene. Framework access holes are permanently filled with composite 1 month after seating.

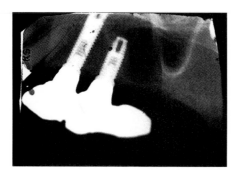

Fig. 6-76

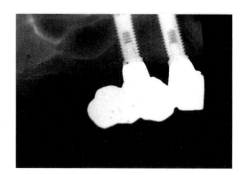

Fig. 6-77

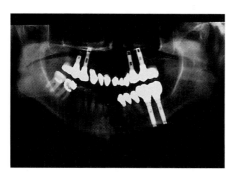

Fig. 6-78

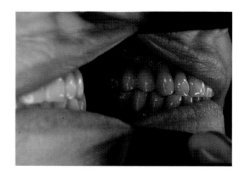

Fig. 6-79

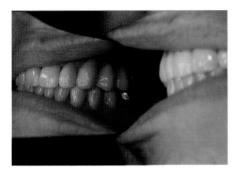

Fig. 6-80

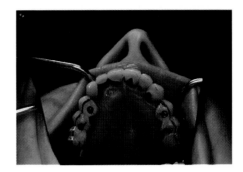

Fig. 6-81

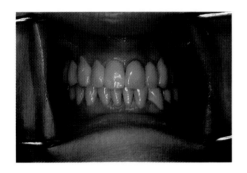

Fig. 6-82

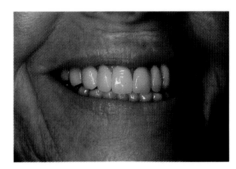

Fig. 6-83

Diverse Abutment Situations

Because of fixture position and angulation, different abutments may be used in combination in prosthesis design. Lack of intermaxillary space may preclude certain abutments because of component height. In these clinical situations a combination of different abutments is necessary for an acceptable prosthetic result. The patient in Fig. 6-84 had four fixtures placed in the maxilla. Loss of natural teeth caused supererup-tion of the opposing mandibular dentition. The distal fixture could not be counter-sunk because of proximity to the maxillary sinus. Fig. 6-85 shows four EsthetiCone abutments in position. A minimum of 6.7 mm of intermaxillary space is necessary to allow for component height. This space is measured from the head of the fixture to the opposing dentition on mounted diagnostic casts. Insufficient space was available for a posterior EsthetiCone abutment. The mandibular crowns were removed, and the occlusal plane was corrected with new crowns. Insufficient space still existed. A UCLA-type abutment that attaches directly to the fixture and needs less space was used. Figs. 6-86 through 6-94 show the procedures from impression technique through the finished prosthetics. A diagnostic wax-up during treatment planning is the ideal procedure if any question about prosthetic design is presented. Diagnostic impressions made directly on the fixtures allow diagnostic waxing and planning for the proper abutment selection. The waxing before abutment selection not only saves time, but also money.

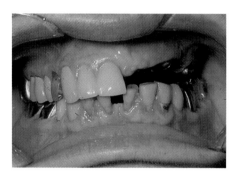

Fig. 6-84

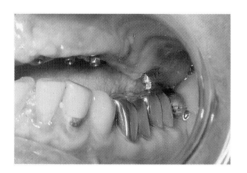

Fig. 6-85

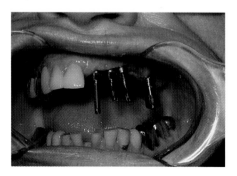

Fig. 6-86

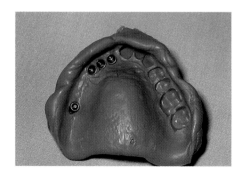

Fig. 6-87

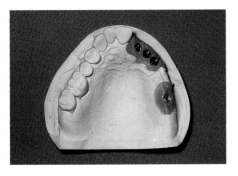

Fig. 6-88

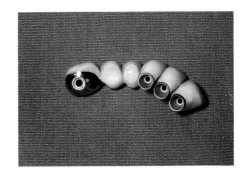

Fig. 6-89

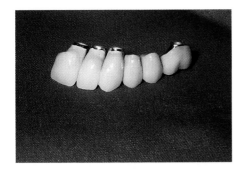

Fig. 6-90

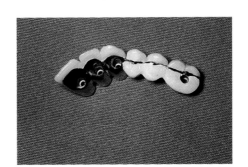

Fig. 6-91

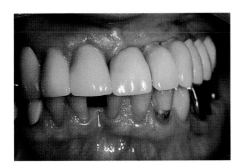

Fig. 6-92

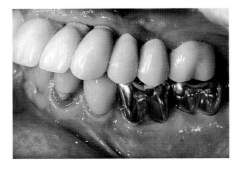

Fig. 6-93

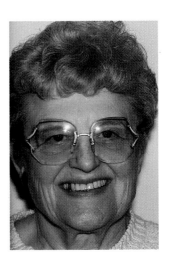

Fig. 6-94

◆ PARTIALLY EDENTULOUS—UCLA PREPS

Less-than-ideal fixture position and angulation may preclude the use of any available abutments in the usual fashion. Modification of the UCLA-type abutment may compensate for esthetic compromise caused by unfavorable fixture position. The patient who is documented had a high smile line complicated by fixture position, which would reveal not only a metal display, but would also prevent adequate access for oral hygiene if the available abutments were used in the typical manner (Figs. 6-95 and 6-96). Fixture angulation is labial, which produced screw access holes exiting through the facial surface of the prosthetics. Sufficient bone is not available for countersinking the fixtures. Ideally, fixtures should be countersunk that place the fixture head at least 4 mm below tissue. This is especially important in the anterior of the maxilla. The angulated abutment allows for the change of the screw access position, but in this case the angulated abutment collar displayed metal supragingivally, thereby compromising esthetics (Figs. 6-97 and 6-98). Modified UCLA abutments are used to allow acceptable esthetics, along with access for oral hygiene.

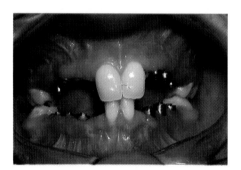

Fig. 6-95

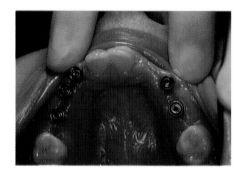

Fig. 6-96

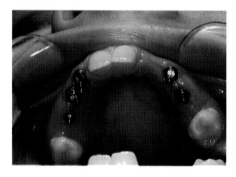

Fig. 6-97

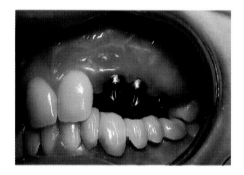

Fig. 6-98

Laboratory

Diagnostic casts from impressions made directly on the fixtures are used to determine abutment design (Fig. 6-99). The anterior abutments are designed as telescopic copings, using antirotational UCLA-type abutments. The copings are placed in position where the natural tooth abutments are located for ideal esthetics.

From the master cast mounting, nonhexed UCLA-type abutments are placed on the two most posterior abutments. The anterior hexed antirotational UCLA-type abutments are designed as telescopic preps. The abutments are reduced in length for bite relationship (Figs. 6-100 and 6-101).

A full contour wax-up is fabricated, and a vinyl polysiloxine matrix is constructed to conform with the facial surfaces, using the antirotational, UCLA-type abutments. Circumferential clearance of the telescopic preps is reverified by repositioning the matrix on the master cast. The telescopic preps are sprued, invested, cast, reclaimed, and then finished with a lapping procedure performed on the inferior surface of the UCLA abutments to ensure accurate interface between the abutment and titanium fixture. The telescopic preps are repositioned into place on the master cast (Figs. 6-102 and 6-103), and the access holes are blocked out with utility wax. A thin coat of wax separator is applied to the preps and surrounding tissue area of the master cast. The matrix is repositioned and held in place with sticky wax. Molten inlay wax is flowed into the matrix and around the preps and is allowed to solidify. Matrix is removed, and the master cast is remounted on the articulator. The bite relationship is verified, and the bridge superstructure is carved and designed, with relieved areas to receive the porcelain application. The bridge superstructure is designed to be cemented on the copings and screwed directly on the posterior fixtures using the antirotational UCLA-type abutments (Fig. 6-104); it is sprued, invested, cast, reclaimed, and finished to the telescopic preps and master cast. The case is returned to the clinic for try-in and accurate fit evaluation.

After clinical evaluation the bridge superstructure is returned to the dental laboratory for porcelain application. Porcelain is applied, contoured, glazed, and finished to the bridge (Figs. 6-105 through 6-108). The completed prostheses are returned to the clinic for insertion delivery to the patient.

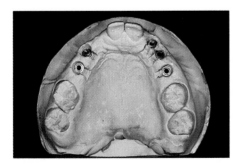

Fig. 6-99

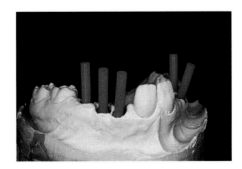

Fig. 6-100

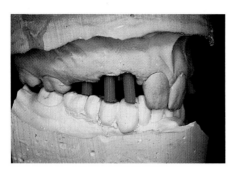

Fig. 6-101

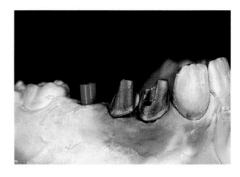

Fig. 6-102

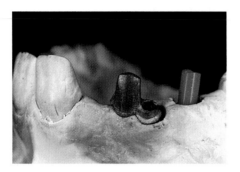

Fig. 6-103

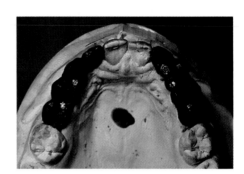

Fig. 6-104

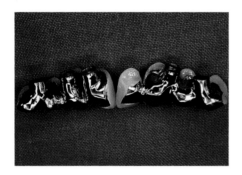

Fig. 6-105

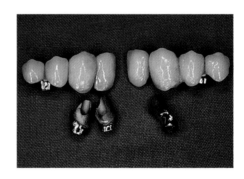

Fig. 6-106

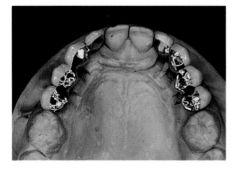

Fig. 6-107

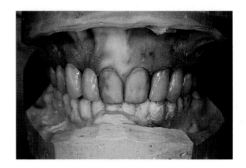

Fig. 6-108

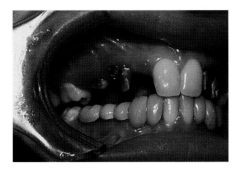

Fig. 6-109

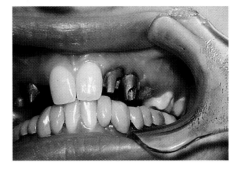

Fig. 6-110

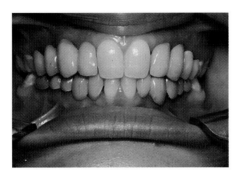

Fig. 6-111

Clinical

Figs. 6-109 and 6-110 show anterior, modified abutments in position clinically. Radiographs are used to verify complete abutment seating on the fixture head. The final prosthetic allows access for oral hygiene. Esthetic compromise caused by the screw access position is eliminated, and metal display is avoided (Fig. 6-111).

7

Overdenture—Implant-Retained Prosthesis

An implant-retained overdenture is an alternative form of treatment to the fixed-implant prosthesis. The overdenture is retained by one of many types of mechanical retention. The denture may attach on a cast bar fixed to the abutments, or it may attach to individual abutments. The patient can remove the overdenture for cleaning. Unconnected abutments and the smaller configuration of the attachment bar (in comparison with the implant prosthesis) allow simplified hygiene protocol.

Patients who have worn conventional dentures for many years and have undergone extensive ridge resorption may require an overdenture to provide acceptable tissue support. The position of the distal-most fixture dictates the cantilever extension with the fixed-implant prosthesis. Patients may not accept the tissue support provided by second premolar or first molar extensions. The overdenture extensions can provide desired tissue support while allowing first or second molar occlusion. Fewer fixtures, abutments, and prosthetic components are required for an overdenture, greatly lowering the cost for treatment. Other advantages include less component stress and breakage and a simplified technique in most situations. When trauma or resorption has diminished the alveolar process in the maxilla, the overdenture may be more esthetic than the implant prosthesis.

Disadvantages include potential movement and irritation from a removable prosthesis or psychological problems associated with a removable prosthesis.

Treatment Planning

Panoramic radiographs and mounted diagnostic casts are made; intraoral, head, and neck examinations are completed; and an in-depth patient interview is performed. During examination, existing dentures are evaluated for vertical dimension of occlusion, lip and cheek support, and esthetics. Models of prosthetic options and pictures or slides of patients with different prosthetic options are shown. The patient's opinion of tissue support, specifically nasiolabial fold, is explored. If the existing labial flange is necessarily thick to compensate for resorption or if the patient's expectations for tissue support include excess support in this area, then an overdenture is indicated, unless a bone graft is used (Figs. 7-1 through 7-3). The buccal corridor and tooth display in the existing prosthesis are evaluated. A patient who shows first or second maxillary molars during maximum smiling may have an unacceptable gap with the fixed-implant prosthesis because of limited cantilever allowed in the maxilla. An

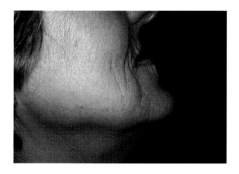

Fig. 7-1

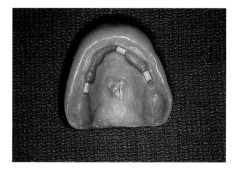

Fig. 7-2

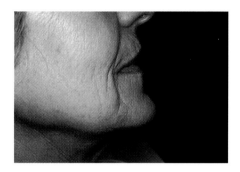

Fig. 7-3

overdenture is indicated in this situation also. After prosthetic evaluation and consultation have occurred, the patient is referred for surgical evaluation. After consultations with the surgeon and the restorative dentist, discussions about the availability of bone for fixture placement, and discussions concerning the patient's expectations in light of financial realities, a decision can be reached concerning prosthetic options.

Mandible

Tissue support in the mental labial fold and external oblique region is evaluated. Patient expectations are discussed. Models of different options are shown, including overdentures with various retentive and financial options, as well as the fixed-implant prosthesis. Pictures of patients with different prosthetic options may be helpful also.

As the patient handles the various models and removes and replaces the dentures, finger strength and dexterity can be evaluated. Examinations, radiographs, records, and surgeon evaluations use the same procedures as those used with the maxillary overdenture.

Overdenture Options

Bar attachment systems
1. Mechanical
   a. Clips
   b. Stud
   c. O-rings
2. Magnetic

Unconnected fixture options
1. Mechanical
   a. Magnetic

The bar attachment system for retaining the overdenture distributes functional force to all fixtures. More retentive options are available with the cast bar. A number of attachments are available, and most work well if used properly. More than one attachment per fixture may be used with a bar system when only one attachment per fixture is possible or if no bar is used to connect fixtures. The bar attachment systems require more components and higher laboratory expense and may be more technique sensitive. Moderate dexterity is necessary for hygiene and placement and removal of the overdenture. Position and number of implants will dictate the length and distal extension of the bar, as well as the number of attachments used. With four or more fixtures the bar may be cantilevered 10 mm distal to the distal-most fixtures, allowing an overdenture, which is mainly implant supported in the mandible. Fewer implants require a combination of tissue and fixture support. In the maxilla, four or more fixtures will allow three or more attachments on the bar and elimination of full palatal coverage. The final denture may have the majority of palatal acrylic removed, leaving the overdenture in a horseshoe configuration.

Procedures—Maxilla and Mandible

Impression procedures are similar to those described for the fixed-implant prosthesis. Preliminary alginate impressions are made 2 weeks following second-stage surgery. The denture is relieved in the area of the abutments and relined with a tissue conditioning material. Custom trays are fabricated with vestibular and palatal extensions similar to a complete denture. The open-window design is used. After complete healing the final impression is made. The titanium hemostats and hexagonal wrench are used to verify abutment tightness. Occasionally, the abutments may appear tight and seated but are not completely seated on the hexagonal head of the fixture. Loosening and retightening the abutment or a radiographic verification can determine the seating. All plaque and calculus are removed from the abutments, and the impression copings are placed (Figs. 7-4 and 7-5). The custom tray is border molded, baseplate wax is used to seal the window, and the tray is placed in the mouth to capture guide pin positions in the wax (Figs. 7-6 and 7-7). After adhesive use the final impression is made. The tray is filled and is seated completely over the guide pins and the impression copings, and border molding is completed (Fig. 7-8). The guide pins are loosened, and the impression is removed. The laboratory replicas are placed, and the impression is poured in diestone as previously described (Figs. 7-9 and 7-10). The attachment and bar extensions are discussed with the laboratory.

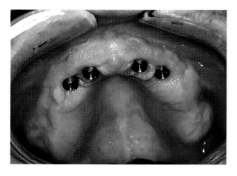

Fig. 7-4

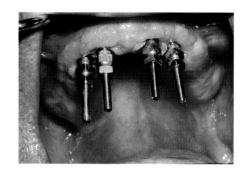

Fig. 7-5

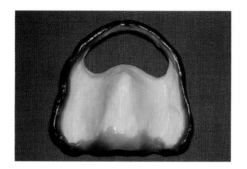

Fig. 7-6

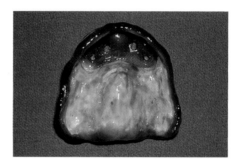

Fig. 7-7

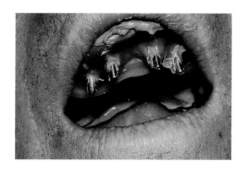

Fig. 7-8

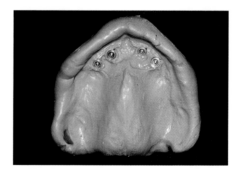

Fig. 7-9

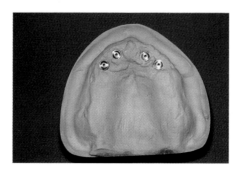

Fig. 7-10

Laboratory Procedures

Depending upon the treatment plan, a variety of clipbar attachments may be considered for the prosthesis, such as a precast clipbar, the Dolder bar, or a plastic custom pattern (Hader bar and CBS System). Additional attachments include stud overdenture attachments, such as Sterngold's ERA, O-SO, and Nobelpharma's ball attachment. Attachments are incorporated into the wax pattern design of the bar, sprued, invested, cast, and reclaimed in the normal manner (Figs. 7-11 through 7-15).

Clinical Trial Fitting

The healing caps are removed, and the abutments are cleaned of all calculus and plaque. The hexagonal wrench is used to tighten the abutments. The attachment bar is passively screwed to place. The framework-abutment interface is checked for accuracy as previously described (Fig. 7-16). The bar is sectioned and soldered if necessary. When an accurate fit exists, a processed base can be made.

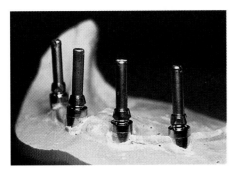

Fig. 7-11

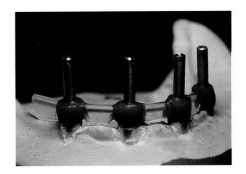

Fig. 7-12

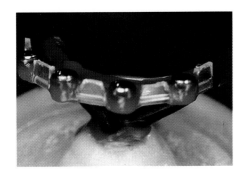

Fig. 7-13

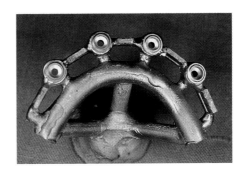

Fig. 7-14

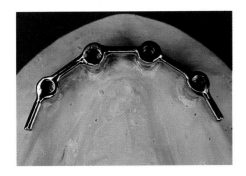

Fig. 7-15

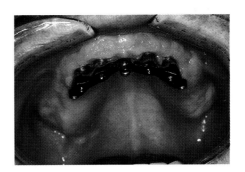

Fig. 7-16

Processed Base

A processed base incorporating attachments provides several advantages when compared with traditional baseplate use. The processed base snaps into the attachment bar, providing stability for interocclusal records. Denture soreness can be adjusted before delivery of the completed prosthesis. Fit and retention from attachments can be perfected before delivery also.

The bar is placed on the master cast with gold screws. Laboratory analogues are placed in each attachment (Figs. 7-17 and 7-18). Fast set plaster is mixed and flowed over the bar, leaving the analogues exposed. The plaster is contoured to completely cover the bar, with no undercuts. The minimum amount of plaster to accomplish this is used. Two thicknesses of baseplate wax are placed onto the master cast (Fig. 7-19), extending over normal denture extensions. The cast is invested in the usual manner and is processed with denture acrylic. After processing occurs, the denture and bar are carefully retrieved from the plaster. The attachment bar is separated from the attachments in the processed base; it is then snapped back into the base to evaluate retention and complete the seating of attachments. The base is trimmed and polished (Fig. 7-20). A wax occlusion rim is then added (Fig. 7-21).

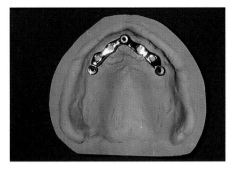

Fig. 7-17

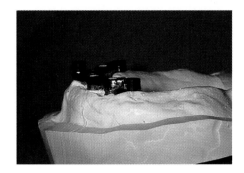

Fig. 7-18

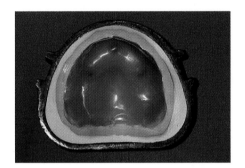

Fig. 7-19

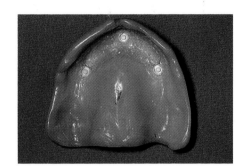

Fig. 7-20

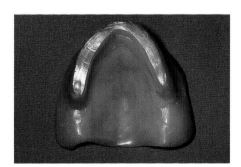

Fig. 7-21

Maxillomandibular Relations

The attachment bar is positioned in the mouth. Pressure indicator paste is placed on the internal area of the processed base and is seated in the mouth. Attachment retention is checked, as is potential denture soreness. If attachments are not seated, denture acrylic in the region of the bar may prevent seating. Examination of the pressure indicator paste pattern and adjustment will allow complete seating. After complete seating has occurred, maxillomandibular relations are completed, establishing lip support and phonetics at the proper vertical dimension of occlusion. Centric relation records and facebow transfer are completed (Figs. 7-22 and 7-23).

The baseplate is mounted on a semiadjustable articulator. Condylar settings are made (if appropriate). Wax contours that are established during maxillomandibular relations are used as guidelines for tooth arrangement.

The bar is secured in the patient's mouth, and the trial tooth arrangement is evaluated (Fig. 7-24). Esthetics, phonetics, and the vertical dimension of occlusion are evaluated. When all parameters are acceptable, another centric relation record is made. Denture soreness can again be adjusted during this appointment.

Laboratory

The denture is processed in the usual manner. After processing, breakout, and laboratory occlusal adjustment have occurred, the overdenture is again snapped into the attachment bar. Occasionally during processing, acrylic may flow into the attachment areas. The acrylic is adjusted again to allow complete seating of the overdenture into the attachment bar. The denture then is polished. The palatal portion of the maxillary denture may be removed if four or more fixtures are present.

Clinical Delivery

The denture is again snapped onto the attachment bar (Figs. 7-25 and 7-26). Pressure indicator paste is used to adjust potential denture soreness. A centric relation record is made, and the denture is remounted in the laboratory for final occlusal refinement. The torque wrench is used to tighten all gold screws to 10 N/cm. Hygiene and homecare instructions are given at this time also.

Mandibular Overdenture Clipbar—Two-Fixture, Tissue-Supported, Using a Precast Nobelpharma Clipbar or a Dolder Bar

From a technical and economical standpoint, several advantages are realized when using this system. Technically speaking the system is one of the least complicated because it is a simple technique involving two solder joints that connect the bar to the gold cylinders. The kit consists of two gold cylinders, two gold screws, a gold bar, and two clip retainers (Fig. 7-27).

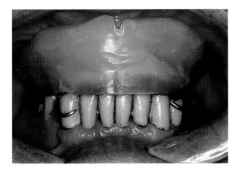

Fig. 7-22

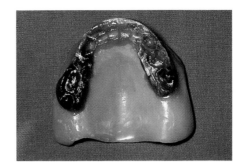

Fig. 7-23

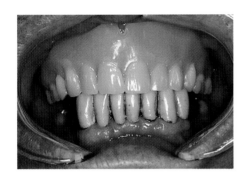

Fig. 7-24

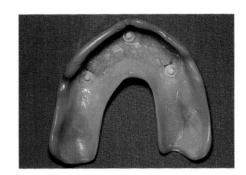

Fig. 7-25

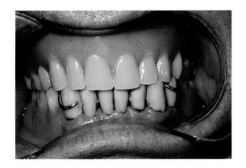

Fig. 7-26

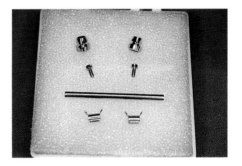

Fig. 7-27

Set-up and Soldering

The gold cylinders are placed onto the abutment replicas and secured in place with guide pin screws (Fig. 7-28). The bar is placed between the two gold cylinders (Fig. 7-29). The precast bar is cut to the required length (Fig. 7-30). The bar is positioned between the cylinders and secured in place with either sticky wax or cyanoacrylate adhesive (Fig. 7-31). The guide pins are unscrewed, and the bar assembly is removed from the master cast and positioned into a soldering investment. Basic soldering techniques are performed using manufacturer's recommended solder (Fig. 7-32). The bar is reclaimed from the investment, cleaned, rubber wheeled, and polished, using protective measures that will not damage the inferior surface of the gold cylinders (Fig. 7-33).

The completed clipbar is returned to the clinic for a try-in to verify accuracy intraorally. An inaccurate fit requires sectioning, indexing, and resoldering the bar (Fig. 7-34).

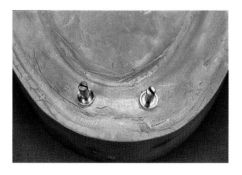

Fig. 7-28

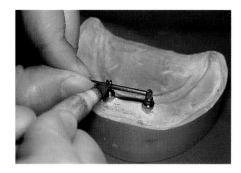

Fig. 7-29

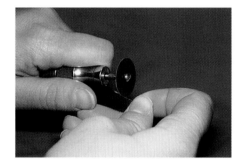

Fig. 7-30

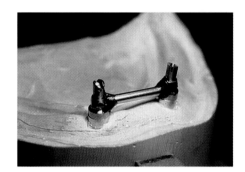

Fig. 7-31

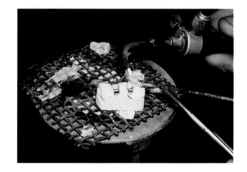

Fig. 7-32

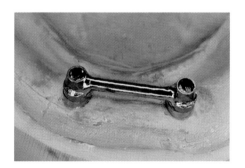

Fig. 7-33

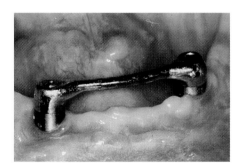

Fig. 7-34

Overdenture Processing to Nobelpharma Clipbar

The clipbar is placed on the master cast and held in position with gold screws. The two retentive clips are evenly spaced on the bar between the gold cylinders (Fig. 7-35). The bar and the gold cylinders are blocked out with dental plaster (Fig. 7-36); the overdenture wax-up is repositioned on the cast, sealed, and processed in the normal manner. The overdenture is finished and polished; clip retention is verified on the master cast (Figs. 7-37 and 7-38) and returned to the clinic for delivery.

◆ MANDIBULAR OVERDENTURE CLIPBAR—PREFABRICATED PLASTIC CLIPBAR PATTERN

A 1 mm thickness of inlay wax is flowed around the retentive surface of gold cylinder. The cylinders are placed on the brass abutment replicas and are held in place with guide pin screws. The distance between abutments is measured and recorded, and the prefabricated plastic bar is cut to proper length. The inferior borders of the plastic bar are trimmed to conform with the topography of the ridge between the fixtures. The bar is aligned with the retromolar pads and is relieved sufficiently so that it does not rest on the tissue, thereby minimizing the possibility of tissue hyperplasia occurring in the future, yet allowing adequate space for hygiene maintenance.

The bar then is secured in position with cyanoacrylate adhesive or sticky wax. Adequate dimension must be maintained for strength in the connecting joints' different proportions.

An indirect spruing technique is the method of preference for this clipbar because it adds rigidity and support for the assembled pattern. An 8-gauge wax sprue is placed on the lingual surface of each gold cylinder. To ensure the integrity of the retentive surface of the bar, a third sprue is attached to the inferior lingual surface of the plastic bar. A 6-gauge plastic wax-coated feeder bar is placed and secured to the sprued bar. Two 6-gauge wax feeder sprues then are attached to the bar, the guide pins are removed, and the assembled sprued pattern is weighed to determine the amount of alloy that will be needed for the casting. The pattern is placed on a sprue former and is vacuum invested, using a phosphate investment. Burnout and casting procedures are performed to manufacturer's directions. The clipbar is cast, reclaimed, cleaned, fit evaluated to the master cast, and prepared for clinical trial fitting.

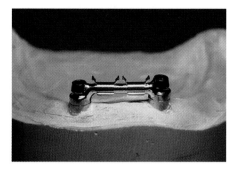

Fig. 7-35

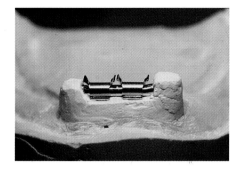

Fig. 7-36

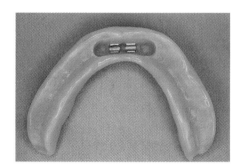

Fig. 7-37

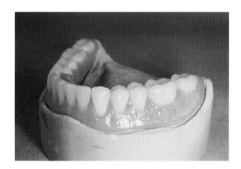

Fig. 7-38

◆ MANDIBULAR OVERDENTURE CLIPBAR
Three- or Four-Fixture Supported

The advantages of the fixture-supported clipbar include the overdenture being secured to the bar at three or four positions, thereby giving at least a tripod retention configuration (Fig. 7-39). This design can produce great stability in the final prosthesis by using either a clipbar, stud attachments, or a combination of the two.

The retentive plastic clip is 5 mm wide; therefore to allow adequate room, a 7 mm to 8 mm plastic pattern is cut for the distal extensions. The distal extended patterns are secured with extreme caution to the gold cylinders, following the crest of the ridge.

An indirect spruing technique is the method of preference for the clipbar, adding rigidity and support for the assembled pattern. An 8-gauge wax sprue is placed on the lingual surface of each gold cylinder. To ensure the integrity of the retentive surface of the bar, a third sprue is attached to the inferior lingual surface of the plastic bar. A 6-gauge, plastic, wax-coated feeder bar is placed and secured to the sprued bar. Two 6-gauge wax feeder sprues are attached to the bar, the guide pins are removed, and the assembled sprued pattern is weighed to determine the amount of alloy required for the casting. The pattern is placed on a sprue former and is vacuum invested, using a high-heat phosphate investment. Burnout and casting procedures are performed to manufacturer's directions.

The clipbar is cast, reclaimed, and cleaned; the fit is evaluated on the master cast. The clipbar is finished, polished, and returned to clinic for a trial fitting.

When the clipbar is returned from the clinic, the overdenture is processed and finished in the usual manner. The completed clipbar and overdenture are returned to the clinic for insertion (Figs. 7-40 through 7-43).

◆ OVERDENTURE CLIPBAR—THREE TO FOUR FIXTURES WITH EXTRA-CORONAL ATTACHMENTS

The fixture-supported overdenture is an alternative to the maxillary and the mandibular fixed bridge. This prosthetic design has a number of advantages. Because of underlying bone resorption the extra bulk in the overdenture creates more facial tissue support. The patient's hygiene maintenance is easier because the removal of the overdenture allows greater access to the fixtures. In some cases the palate in the maxillary overdenture may be removed to enable the patient to have a greater thermal sensitivity.

Clinical

The impressions for the clipbars are taken in the usual manner with open-windowed custom trays. Impression copings and guide pins are placed, and the tissue is impressed, using vinyl polysiloxane impression material. Clinical and laboratory procedures are similar to those shown in Figs. 7-4 through 7-26.

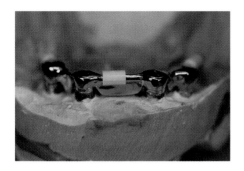

Fig. 7-39

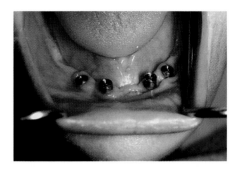

Fig. 7-40

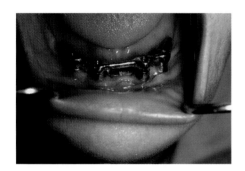

Fig. 7-41

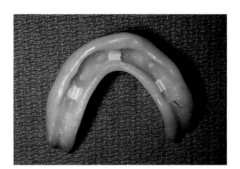

Fig. 7-42

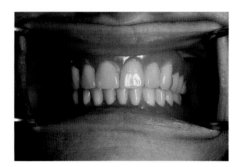

Fig. 7-43

Laboratory Procedures

The master casts are poured and mounted on a semiadjustable articulator, using the intraoral bite registrations. The gold cylinders are secured to the abutment replicas with guide pin screws. Inlay wax is placed around each gold cylinder, and wax is flowed to connect each of the cylinders, forming a wax bar.

Two ERA extracoronal attachments and two O-SO attachments are affixed to the bar waxing, using a surveyor for parallelism. The two extracoronal attachments are placed distal to the posterior abutments on the crest of the ridge. When waxing the inferior surfaces, adjacent space must be allowed for proper hygiene.

On the mandible (Figs. 7-44 through 7-49), two ERA extracoronal attachments, along with two O-S O-rings, are used. The O-SO attachments were chosen because of the lack of distance they have between the abutments. This distance does not allow for ERAs or clipbar design.

Waxing is similar to that stated previously for the clipbar procedures, with the parallel placement of the O-SO attachments on the superior surface (as shown).

The wax patterns are indirectly sprued and cast in a normal fashion. Castings are reclaimed and reverified to the master cast.

Castings are sent to the clinic for intraoral fit evaluation. They are verified passively and secured with gold screws. The interfaces between the gold cylinders and the abutments are examined for accuracy of fit. If any discrepancies are noted the bar is cut, soldering indexes are made, and the framework is returned to the laboratory for soldering. If no changes are to be made to the framework, it is returned to the laboratory for a final polishing and processing of the overdentures.

Overdentures are processed using recommended manufacturer's directions for processing stud attachments.

Unconnected Fixtures

Many attachments have been manufactured for fabricating implant-retained overdentures without using an attachment bar. The attachments are designed to connect directly to the abutment. There are fewer components, less clinical and laboratory time is used; therefore, fees are lower, making this an economic alternative to an attachment bar–retained overdenture. Impressions, try-ins, records, and procedures are identical, except that bar fabrication is eliminated. A processed acrylic base allows for a more secure clinical record making.

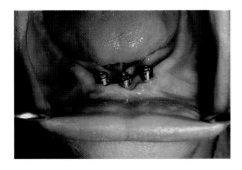

Fig. 7-44

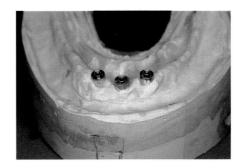

Fig. 7-45

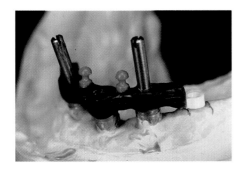

Fig. 7-46

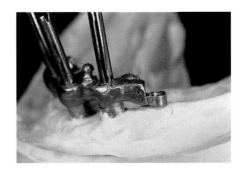

Fig. 7-47

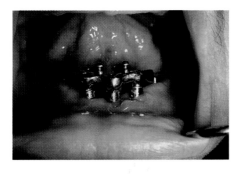

Fig. 7-48

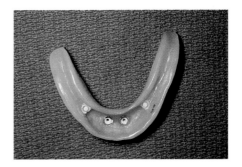

Fig. 7-49

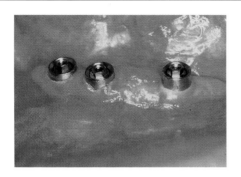

Fig. 7-50

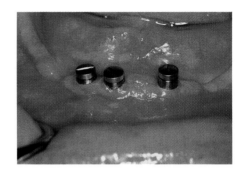

Fig. 7-51

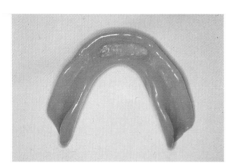

Fig. 7-52

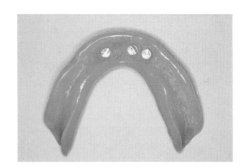

Fig. 7-53

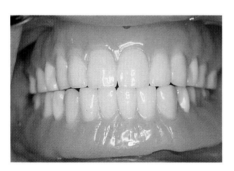

Fig. 7-54

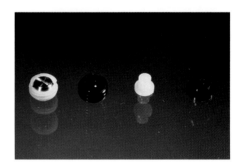

Fig. 7-55

◆ MAGNETIC ATTACHMENTS

The development of rare-earth element magnets has greatly increased the magnetic force available for prosthetic retention in a clinically applicable size. Magnetic systems incorporate the magnet, which is either a neodymium-iron-boron alloy or a samarium-cobalt alloy. Both alloys corrode quickly in oral fluids and must be encased in a protective coating to prevent contamination and loss of magnetism. The second part of the magnet system is the ferromagnetic keeper (Figs. 7-50 and 7-51). This component is designed to screw onto the abutment and is made of a ferro-magnetic alloy. The magnet is retained in the denture.

The magnets experience loss of magnetism when exposed to the heat of processing; therefore a plastic magnet analogue (if available) must be used until processing has been completed. The magnets can be picked up with autopolymerizing resin at the delivery appointment (Figs. 7-52 through 7-54). The Shriner magnet system has a series of laboratory analogues that allow processed base fabrications, as well as processing with magnet analogues (Fig. 7-55). The magnet analogues are unscrewed, and the plastic-encased magnets are screwed in at the delivery appointment.

Magnetic systems have shown problems involving corrosion (as previously mentioned). Even with a metal or a plastic encasement, the forces of mastication can wear through the encasement. Corrosion and rapid loss of magnetism occur once the encasement is broken.

8

Special Cases

This chapter will demonstrate unique applications for fixture-retained prosthetics. Clinical and laboratory techniques for most cases are beyond the scope of this text; however, the text displays a variety of applications that can lead to a better quality of life-style for persons with the following particular defects.

Maxillary Fixed Prostheses

An implant-retained overdenture provides a functional and esthetic result for patients and at the same time halts bone resorption. Many patients desire an implant-retained prosthesis that will eliminate all removable designs. Psychologically, this enhances the prosthetic acceptance by returning the patient to as normal a life-style and mastication as possible. A fixed prosthesis rehabilitates the patient to resemble the way he or she looked before any tooth loss occurred.

A high smile line may reveal at least the first maxillary molar. Cantilever restrictions in the maxilla allow a 10 mm maximum extension distal to the distal-most fixture. Often, inadequate bone exists inferior to the maxillary sinus for fixture placement. Patients desiring an implant-retained fixed prosthesis may have an esthetic compromise because of limited cantilever and second premolar occlusion. Occasionally, adequate bone exists in the pterygoid plate region for fixture placement. With fixtures in this region patients can be given 12 to 14 teeth on the implant prosthesis and will experience no compromise in esthetics. The cantilevered section of the prosthesis is eliminated also, reducing forces transmitted to implant components.

The patient in Fig. 8-1 desired a fixed maxillary prosthesis. For her, an overdenture was not an acceptable alternative. Bone grafting was planned to ensure a fixed prosthesis. Adequate bone was found in the pterygoid plate region bilaterally for fixture placement. Seven fixtures were placed (Fig. 8-2). This fixture placement allowed the fabrication of a fixed prosthesis, and bone grafting procedures were not necessary (Figs. 8-3 through 8-5). For esthetic purposes the dental laboratory designed and applied pink porcelain on the maxillary anterior to match the gingival tissue (Fig. 8-6). A high smile line that displays first molars is seen in the finished prosthetic result (Figs. 8-7 and 8-8).

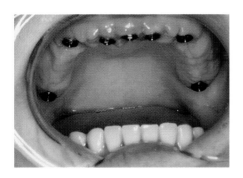

Fig. 8-1

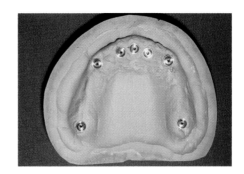

Fig. 8-2

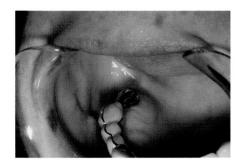

Fig. 8-3

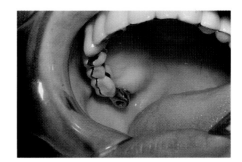

Fig. 8-4

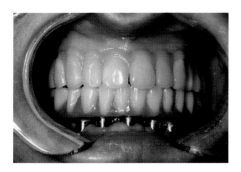

Fig. 8-5

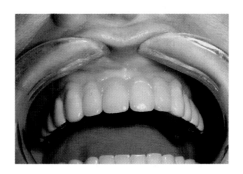

Fig. 8-6

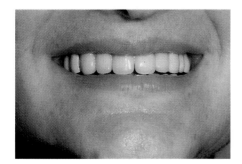

Fig. 8-7

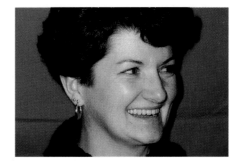

Fig. 8-8

Bone Grafting

Severe bone resorption, trauma, congenital defects, or tumor removal may leave inadequate bone for fixture placement. Bone grafts harvested from the iliac crest and other sites can be used to provide bone for fixture placement and to augment tissue contours to enhance the esthetics of the prosthetic result (Figs. 8-9 and 8-10).

The patient shown in Fig. 8-11 was adamant about receiving a fixed prosthesis in the maxilla. A full onlay bone graft was placed and secured with six Branemark fixtures. Additional fixtures were placed in the pterygoid plate region bilaterally. A fixed prosthesis was possible because the bone graft allowed fixture placement and augmented buccal tissue contours (Figs. 8-12 through 8-16).

The patient shown in Fig. 8-17 desired a fixed maxillary prosthesis, also. Anterior maxillary resorption caused by opposing natural dentition left insufficient bone for anterior fixture placement. Bone was harvested from the patient's chin and was grafted to the nasal floor (Figs. 8-17 and 8-18). Five fixtures were placed in the maxilla, and a fixed prosthesis was fabricated (Figs. 8-19 through 8-26).

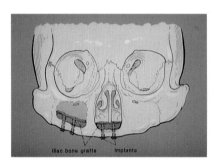

Fig. 8-9

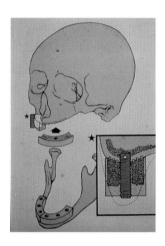

Fig. 8-10

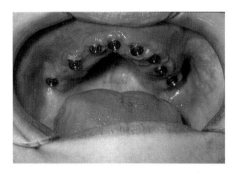

Fig. 8-11

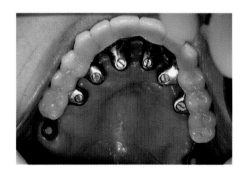

Fig. 8-12

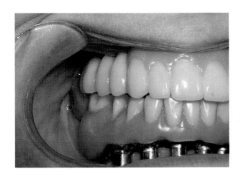

Fig. 8-13

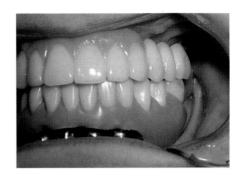

Fig 8-14

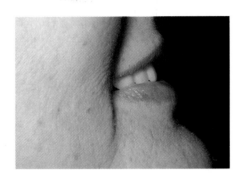

Fig. 8-15

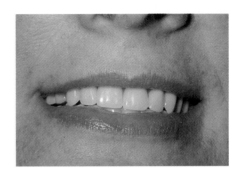

Fig. 8-16

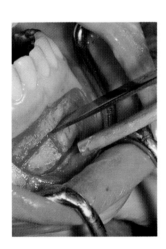

Fig. 8-17

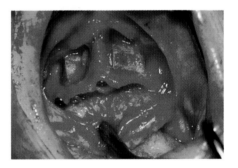

Fig. 8-18

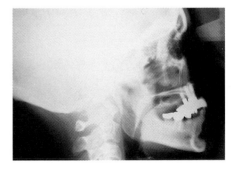

Fig. 8-19

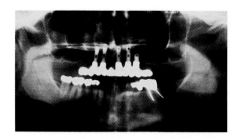

Fig. 8-20

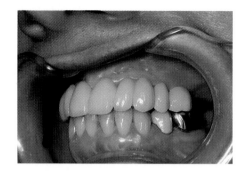

Fig. 8-21

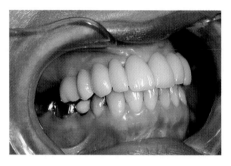

Fig. 8-22

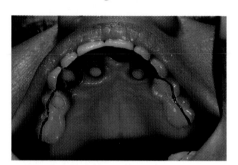

Fig. 8-23

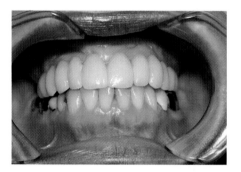

Fig. 8-24

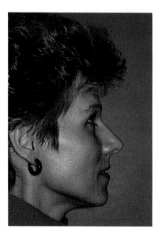

Fig. 8-25

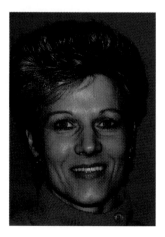

Fig. 8-26

Bone Grafting—Oncologic Defects

The patient in Figs. 8-27 and 8-28 had resections for ameloblastoma at ages 3 weeks and 6 months. Treatment partials were worn by the patient until the age of 18 years. Radiographs of the anatomical defect can be seen in Figs. 8-29 and 8-30. Bone was harvested from the iliac crest and grafted on the maxillary defect. Three fixtures were placed in the graft (Figs. 8-31 and 8-32). The finished prosthesis is seen in Figs. 8-32 through 8-37.

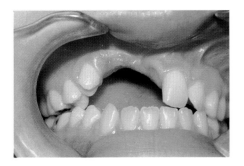

Fig. 8-27

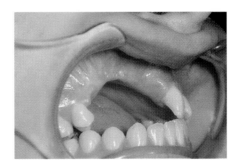

Fig. 8-28

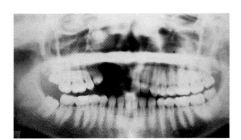

Fig. 8-29

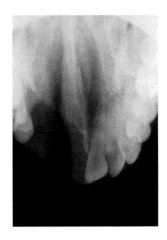

Fig. 8-30

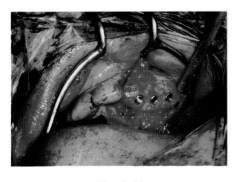

Fig. 8-31

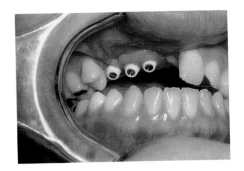

Fig. 8-32

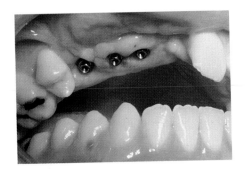

Fig. 8-33

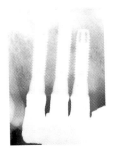

Fig. 8-34

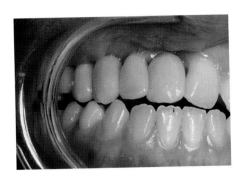

Fig. 8-35

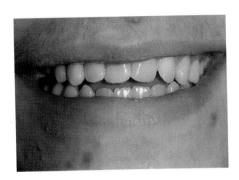

Fig. 8-36

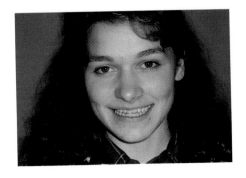

Fig. 8-37

Mandibular Split Frame Prosthesis

Psychologic reaction to fixture placement and the procedures of osseointegration is analyzed when the clinician plans the treatment. Another patient received a traditional hybrid mandibular fixed prosthesis. Three millimeters of metalwork were visible above the mandibular gingiva when the lower lip was fully retracted. During speech and smiling the abutments were never visible; however, the patient had a hysterical reaction to the presence of abutments. A split frame prosthesis was designed to provide a superstructure that would cover the abutments and could be removed for hygiene during clinical visits.

This design was first introduced by Patrick Henry, D.D.S., to compensate for fixtures that were to be placed or angled buccally. Two plastic dovetail (PD) attachments were placed horizontally and parallel to each other on the superior surface of the framework. Screw holes were tapped into the distal extension region of the inferior framework to secure the superior section of the prosthesis (Fig. 8-38).

The superior framework was then designed and fabricated, incorporating the male PD attachments to slide horizontally and to engage the inferior framework. A plastic sleeve was waxed into the superior framework to allow access to the set screw that was used to secure the superior portion of the prosthesis. The finished split frame prosthesis is seen in Figs. 8-39 through 8-42.

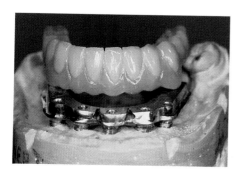

Fig. 8-38

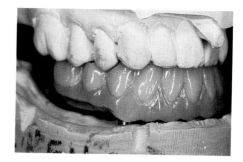

Fig. 8-39

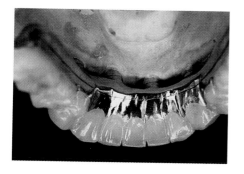

Fig. 8-40

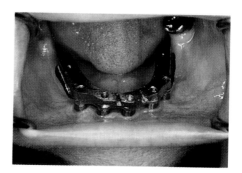

Fig. 8-41

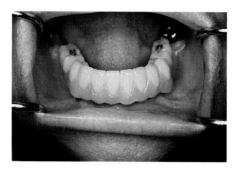

Fig. 8-42

Acquired and Congenital Defects

Cleft palate patients and patients who have had surgical resections for tumor removal may have anatomic defects that require prosthetic replacement. Traditional prosthetics necessitate the use of existing teeth or other anatomy for retaining the prosthesis. The lack of retention for prosthetics often leaves the patient severely compromised functionally. Fixture placement provides much greater retention for prosthetics, improving speech and other functions (Fig. 8-43).

Maxillectomy Defects

The patient in Fig. 8-44 has a left maxillectomy caused by squamous cell carcinoma. She had worn an edentulous obturator for 20 years, with little success. Her speech was hypernasal. Food and liquids leaked out of her nose during deglutition. Three fixtures were placed in the remaining maxillary alveolus. A framework was made that incorporated three ERA coronal attachments (Figs. 8-45 and 8-46). An obturator was fabricated that engaged the attachment bar (Figs. 8-47 through 8-49). The fixture-retained prosthesis gave the patient much better function. Her ability to eat a proper diet was enhanced, and her speech was greatly improved.

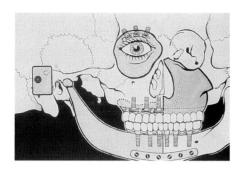

Fig. 8-43

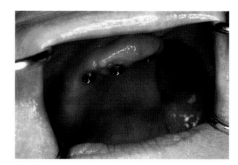

Fig. 8-44

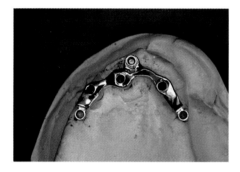

Fig. 8-45

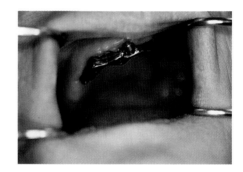

Fig. 8-46

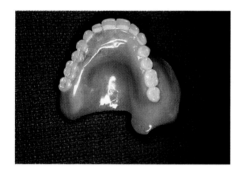

Fig. 8-47

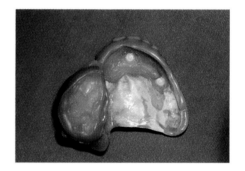

Fig. 8-48

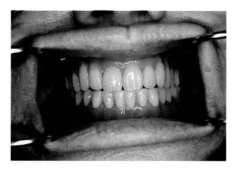

Fig. 8-49

Cleft Palate Rehabilitation

Cleft palate patients have functional defects that are similar to those of the maxillectomy patient. Fixture-retained prosthetics improve all oral functions, including speech, chewing, and swallowing. The patient in Fig. 8-50 had seven fixtures placed to support an attachment bar that could incorporate CEKA coronal attachments (Figs. 8-51 and 8-52). The obturator encompassed the male portion of the attachment system (Figs. 8-53 and 8-54). The finished prosthesis is seen in Fig. 8-55.

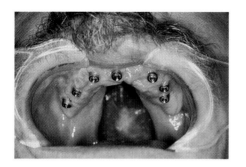

Fig. 8-50

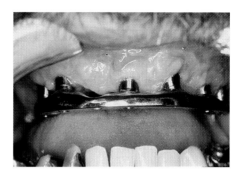

Fig. 8-51

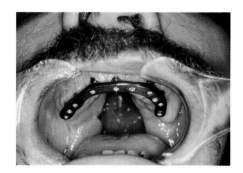

Fig. 8-52

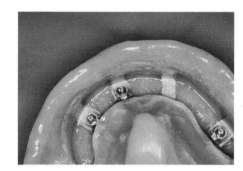

Fig. 8-53

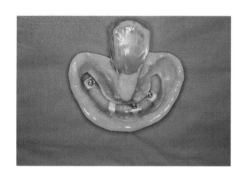

Fig. 8-54

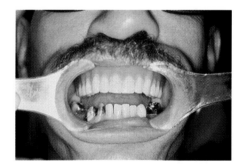

Fig. 8-55

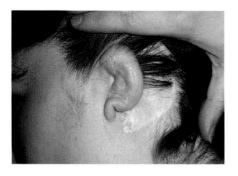

Fig. 8-56

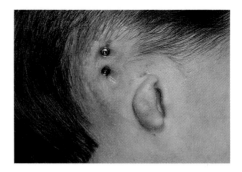

Fig. 8-57

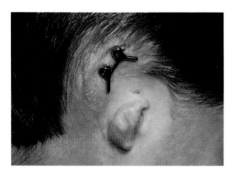

Fig. 8-58

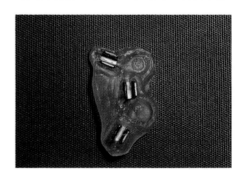

Fig. 8-59

Craniofacial Prosthetics

Bone outside the oral cavity has capabilities for osseointegration similar to those of intraoral bone. Patients with acquired or congenital craniofacial defects can benefit from fixture placement, also. Plastic surgery provides the ideal reconstruction to correct anatomic defects; however, it has its limits as far as esthetic replacement for craniofacial defects is concerned. Fig. 8-56 shows auricular reconstruction after eight surgical procedures. Prosthetic replacements provide a more esthetic result. Scarring and pain from multiple grafting procedures are eliminated by using fixture-retained prosthetics.

The patient in Fig. 8-57 has hemifacial microsomia. The right ear remnant is seen in relation to fixture position. Three fixtures were integrated, but only two were used because the third fixture was in the hairline and was not essential for retention. Impressions were made, and a gold bar was fabricated, using traditional components (Fig. 8-58). An acrylic framework was used to house three gold clips (Fig. 8-59). The ear was waxed on the master cast, incorporating the acrylic matrix with clips. The ear was invested, and intrinsically stained silicone was processed in the mold (Fig. 8-60). The finished auricular prosthesis is seen in Figs. 8-61 through 8-63.

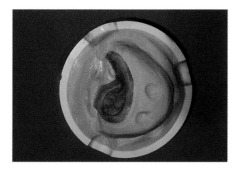

Fig. 8-60

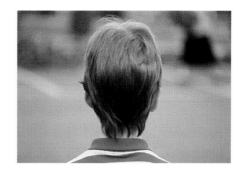

Fig. 8-61

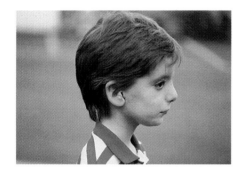

Fig. 8-62

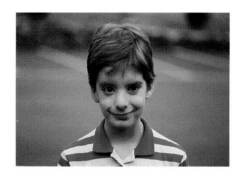

Fig. 8-63

Extrinsic staining was completed before prosthetic delivery. The fixture-retained prosthesis has several advantages over an adhesive-retained prosthesis. Stability and retention are greatly increased with clip bar retention. Athletic pursuits are possible without dislodging the prosthesis. Patients who desire to wear an earring can do so without worrying about the ear falling off. The use of adhesives and the daily cleaning of a normal prosthesis wear down borders, and the tinting may be distorted; whereas the fixture-retained auricular prosthesis may last several more years without replacement. The fixture-retained craniofacial prosthesis greatly enhances the patient's quality of life.

CHAPTER

9

Complications

Implant prosthodontics can be straightforward when fixture position and angulation are ideal. If prosthetic components are used properly and if framework design and fit are perfect, complications can be minimized. Component and framework breakage, inadequate tissue support, poor fixture position and angulation, and fixture loss complicate prosthetic treatment and may compromise the final prosthetic result. The purpose of this chapter is to discuss complications with implant rehabilitation and possible causes and solutions for the complications.

Component and Framework Design

The reasons for gold and abutment screw loosening and fracture are listed below:

1. Screw design
2. Inadequate torque application
3. Cantilever extension
4. Inaccurate framework abutment interface
5. Occlusal discrepancy and jaw relationship
6. Fixture position and arch form

Screw Design

A conical screw was originally used for framework retention (Fig. 9-1). These screws had a tendency to loosen. Torque applied through handheld screwdrivers was used for tightening. Hand strength varies between dentists, and incomplete tightening or binding on the conical screw head caused occasional loosening of the screws and, therefore, the prosthesis. An increase in prosthesis movement applied torque to implant components and contributed to component loosening and breakage. The gold screw and gold cylinder have been redesigned, and a flathead screw is now used. The force of torquing the screw is now incorporated into the threads, and the inadvertent loosening of properly torqued flathead screws is rare (Fig. 9-2). These screws are weaker than the conical screws, and excessive hand torquing can induce stress fractures or actually fracture the screws.

Inadequate Torque Application

A mechanical torque driver has been developed to ensure proper tightening (Figs. 9-3 and 9-4). Recommended torque for gold screws is 10 Ncm, and 20 Ncm is recommended for the abutment screw. A manual torque converter is available to adjust torque between 10 Ncm and 20 Ncm. Another torque driver has been developed

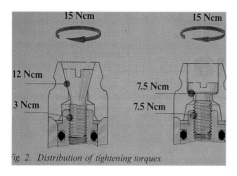

Fig. 9-1

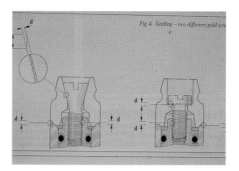

Fig. 9-2

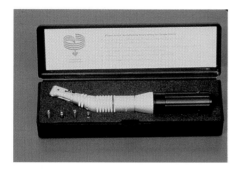

Fig. 9-3

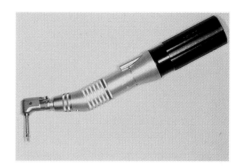

Fig. 9-4

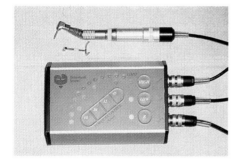

Fig. 9-5

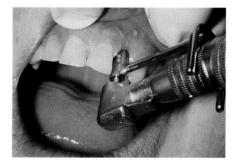

Fig. 9-6

that is electric and is adjustable to 32 Ncm for the CeraOne system, 20 Ncm for abutment screws, and 10 Ncm for gold screws (Figs. 9-5 and 9-6). It is recommended that all screws be tightened with one of the torque drivers. Patients are advised at the prosthetic delivery appointment and during hygiene recall appointments to monitor for prosthesis loosening. Abutments with a visual framework abutment interface are checked for looseness by observing the interface while grasping the incisors and attempting to move the prosthesis. If movement is present, saliva can be seen percolating at the interface. If movement is suspected, the patient is instructed to call for an appointment immediately. If movement is detectable clinically, the gold screws are accessed and checked for tightness. The prosthesis is removed, and all components are examined. If any of the gold screws are loose, all of the gold screws should be replaced. Undetectable stress fractures may be present in previously used screws if prosthesis movement is present. Broken gold on abutment screws may be evident when the prosthesis is removed (Figs. 9-7 through 9-9). The remaining shaft is removed from the abutment screw by using hemostats if adequate length exists for engagement. An explorer tip that is used in a counterclockwise direction on the screw shaft also may work. A slowly rotating #0.5 bur or a #1 round bur in a slow speed handpiece is used for shafts that are broken close to the abutment screw head. When a loose prosthesis is removed, abutment screws may be fractured. The junction of the abutment screw head and shaft is where fracture usually occurs. The same methods for gold screw removal are used for abutment screw shaft removal. Individual abutment screws are available and are used with the original abutment, unless it has been damaged; this will ensure that the old prosthesis will fit the same as it did before the screw fractured. If total abutment replacement is necessary, the same length abutment is used, the original prosthesis is positioned, and the interfaces are checked (as previously described). Rarely, the gold screw slot may be distorted by repeated loosening and tightening, preventing removal of the screw. The screw head can be reslotted, if accessible, or the head of the screw can be severed to the shank with a dental bur (Figs. 9-10 through 9-12).

Cantilever Extension

The cantilevered distance beyond the distal fixtures determines the lever arm length and the amount of force that is transmitted to the fixtures, framework, and components. Twenty millimeters of cantilever were originally recommended for the fixed mandibular prosthesis on four or more implants. Several factors may modify cantilever length, including fixture length, fixture arch form, fixture spacing, bone quality, occlusal considerations, and parafunctional habits. More research is needed to determine cantilever length for each situation. It is recommended that the cantilever length on five or more fixtures in the mandible be limited to 15 mm or less and 10 mm or less in the maxilla when five or more fixtures are used. The modifying factors listed above may shorten the recommended distance of cantilever.

Overextension of the cantilever may lead to gold screw fracture, abutment screw fracture, loosening of the prosthesis, and possibly fixture loss. If an existing prosthesis has an intimately fitting framework (no occlusal discrepancies and no parafunctional habits exist) but component fracture occurs repeatedly, the cantilever length should be shortened.

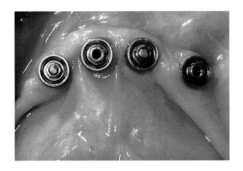

Fig. 9-7

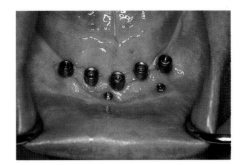

Fig. 9-8

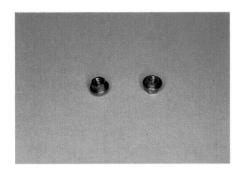

Fig. 9-9

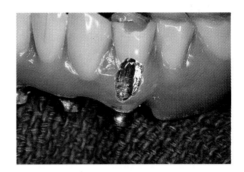

Fig. 9-10

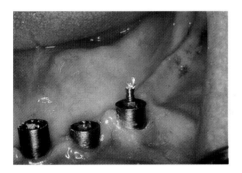

Fig. 9-11

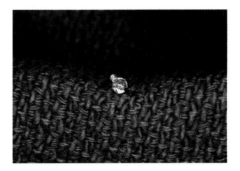

Fig. 9-12

Inaccurate Framework Abutment Interface

The prosthetic components are designed to specific tolerances to allow a precise junction between abutments and prosthetic frameworks. An ideal framework abutment connection is one that has circumferential contact with no opening at the interface. Inaccuracy in framework abutment interface will cause a constant tension on components when the gold screws are tightened to recommended torque. This constant stress may cause component loosening or breakage. Fixtures under tension may be sensitive for the patient, and ill-fitting frameworks may eventually cause loss of osseointegration. Therefore, the framework abutment connection must be passive for long-term success. When evaluating the fit, screws should be tightened one at a time, while observing the lift of the frame and the open interfaces. Torquing all the gold screws before evaluating the interface may bend the framework, giving the appearance of accuracy. Figs. 9-13 through 9-16 show reasonable visual interfacing; however, when the distal screws are loosened, the gap between the framework and the abutment opens significantly. If these frames are seated, a constant stress is placed on the fixtures and the components, potentially causing complications. Therefore, all framework fittings should be visualized before tightening all screws. Individual screws should be tightened, and the framework fit should be observed on other abutments. *ANY* discrepancy in fit demands framework sectioning, solder indexing, soldering, and then a clinical reevaluation of the fit.

Occlusal Factors

Optimally, occlusal force should be shared equally by all fixtures. Although an equal distribution is rarely achieved, force distribution can be improved with careful occlusal adjustment during laboratory remounts, as well as intraorally during the delivery appointment. Shimstock is used to verify all occlusal contacts. In a Class II jaw relationship or with the fixture angled or placed lingual to the ridge crest, an anterior cantilever may be present along with the distal cantilever (Fig. 9-17); this will transmit additional force to the components, and an increase in component breakage may be seen.

Framework Fracture

Properly designed framework should not fracture. A cross-sectional dimension of at least 4 mm 3 6 mm is needed. A J-shaped beam, with the occlusal gingival height having the greater dimension, will provide strength and resist fracture. The alloy should have a tensile strength of at least 60,000. Common areas of framework fracture are through the solder joints and just distal to the distal-most fixture (Figs. 9-18 through 9-26). Because of the cantilever this region is subjected to a higher force, and an adequate cross-sectional dimension is needed to resist fracture. Improperly soldered joints also are subject to fracture (Figs. 9-18 through 9-22). Fractured solder joints may be reindexed intraorally and then soldered. The heat of soldering will destroy any acrylic veneering material; this is replaced after the framework fit has been verified after soldering. Framework fracture caused by a minimal cross-sectional dimension in the metal may require a frame remake.

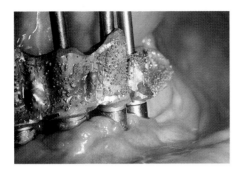

Fig. 9-13

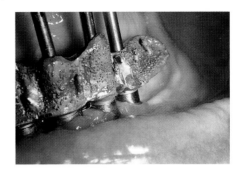

Fig. 9-14

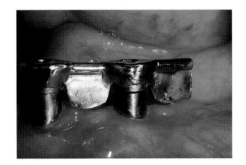

Fig. 9-15

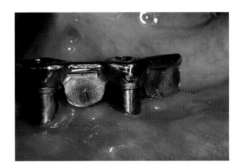

Fig. 9-16

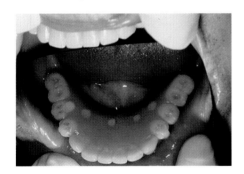

Fig. 9-17

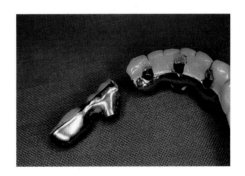

Fig. 9-18

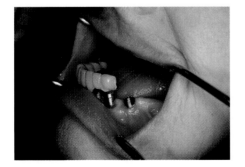

Fig. 9-19

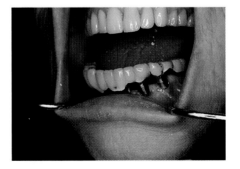

Fig. 9-20

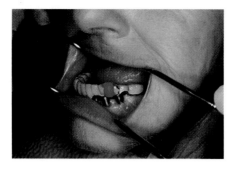

Fig. 9-21

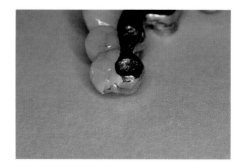

Fig. 9-22

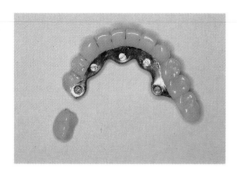

Fig. 9-23

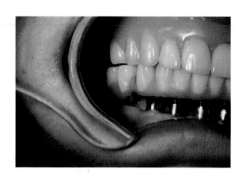

Fig. 9-24

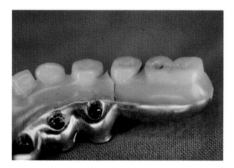

Fig. 9-25

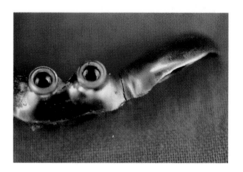

Fig. 9-26

Tissue Support

Alveolar resorption or trauma may leave an inadequate amount of alveolar bone, thereby leaving patients with an inadequate tissue contour to support an implant-retained prosthesis. Complete dentures compensate for bone loss, with the denture flange providing tissue support. Patients wearing conventional prosthetics may be accustomed to ideal or excess tissue support provided by the flange, especially in the mentolabial fold and nasolabial fold. An implant-supported fixed prosthesis may not provide tissue support or esthetically acceptable contours in these areas. The alternatives for use in the mandible are an implant-retained overdenture and a gingival insert (Figs. 9-27 through 9-30). In the maxilla, bone grafting may provide ideal contours. An overdenture or gingival insert may esthetically compensate for bone loss. The overdenture technique is described in Chapter 7.

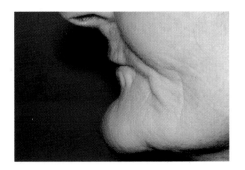

Fig. 9-27

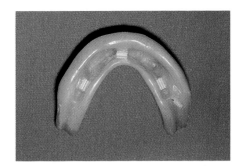

Fig. 9-28

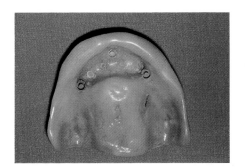

Fig. 9-29

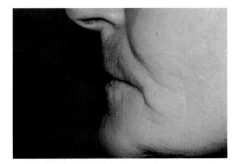

Fig. 9-30

Gingival Insert

The insert is made by making an impression of the completed fixed prosthesis. A polyvinyl siloxane putty is mixed and placed in the labial vestibule. It should cover the labial side of the prosthesis to the floor of the vestibule. The material should be pressed between the abutments and should cover the distal buccal extent of the prosthesis. After the material has set, the putty matrix is removed. Injection viscosity polyvinyl siloxane impression material is placed in a thin layer on the lingual surface of the putty, and the matrix is positioned back in the mouth. The impression is removed after it has set and is cast in diestone (Fig. 9-31 and 9-32). A wax pattern is made on the master cast (Fig. 9-33). The cast is invested, boiled out, and may be packed with a soft reline material or methylmethacrylate resin (Figs. 9-34 through 9-37). The cast will be destroyed with the methylmethacrylate resin, and a duplicate cast that is made before investing is used for adjustments and for a proper path of insertion.

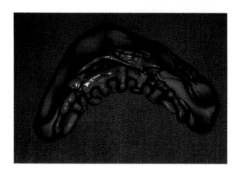

Fig. 9-31

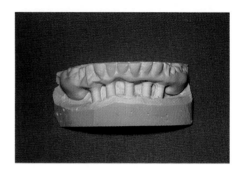

Fig. 9-32

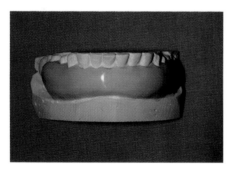

Fig. 9-33

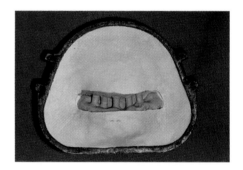

Fig. 9-34

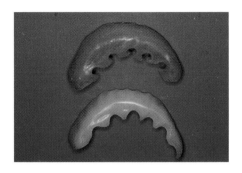

Fig. 9-35

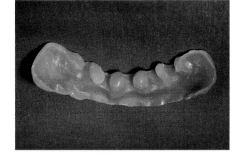

Fig. 9-36

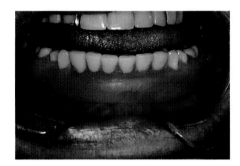

Fig. 9-37

Fixture Position and Angulation

Poor planning, lack of adequate bone, or poor surgical technique may leave fixtures and abutments in a less-than-ideal position. Esthetics, phonetics, hygiene, and prosthetic design may be compromised by poor implant position (Figs. 9-38 through 9-42). In severe cases, the implants may not be usable at all and may have to be removed or left in the bone without abutment placement. Components have been developed that compensate for poor implant angulation (Figs. 9-42 through 9-46). The angulated abutment was designed to change the abutment angle by 30 degrees. In turn this changes the screw access direction by 30 degrees. This change in angulation eliminates prosthetic compromise in most situations.

The angulated abutment has 12 facets and 12 positions of angulation in a 360 degree circle. It is recommended that the prosthodontist place the angulated abutment to ensure the best possible angulation (Figs. 9-47 and 9-48). A system of impression copings, gold cylinders, laboratory analogues, and healing caps have been developed for use with the angulated abutment.

Labially tipped abutments may have a screw access hole that exits through the labial veneering material or through the incisal edge; this compromises the strength and esthetics of the veneer. Excess labial angulation and position may interfere with normal denture flange position with an implant retained overdenture (Figs. 9-49 through 9-51). Lingual or palatal angulation may encroach on the neutral zone and interfere with speech (Figs. 9-52 and 9-53).

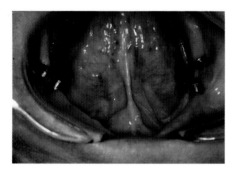

Fig. 9-38

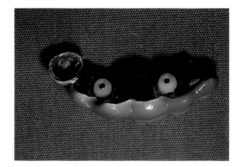

Fig. 9-39

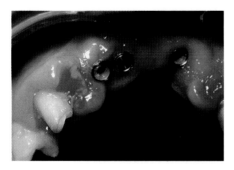

Fig. 9-40

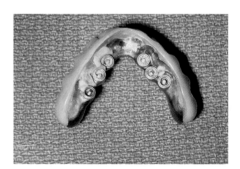

Fig. 9-41

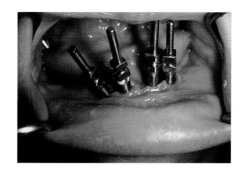

Fig. 9-42

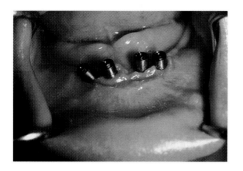

Fig. 9-43

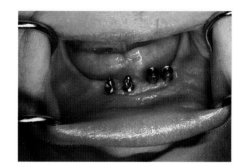

Fig. 9-44

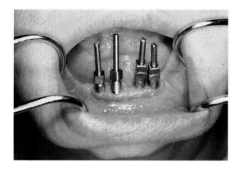

Fig. 9-45

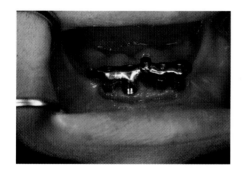

Fig. 9-46

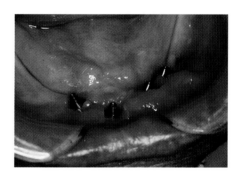

Fig. 9-47

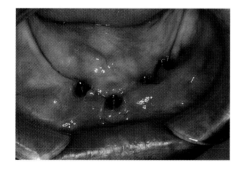

Fig. 9-48

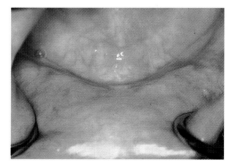

Fig. 9-49

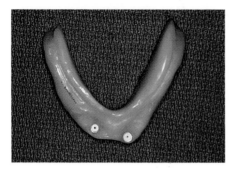

Fig. 9-50

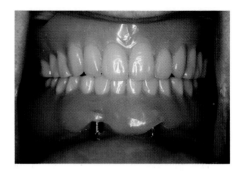

Fig. 9-51

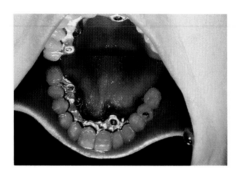

Fig. 9-52

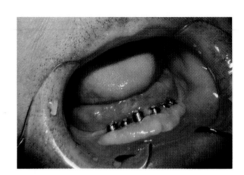

Fig. 9-53

Clinical Procedure

In the maxillary anterior the collar of the angulated abutment may compromise esthetics or oral hygiene (Figs. 9-54 through 9-58). This problem can be minimized if adequate bone exists for countersinking the fixture enough to have the abutment collar below tissue. Most angulation and position problems can be eliminated by careful treatment planning and communication between the restorative dentist, the oral surgeon, and the dental technician, as well as by the use of a surgical stent.

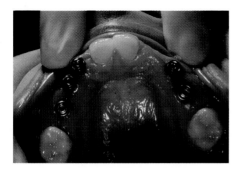

Fig. 9-54

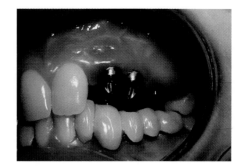

Fig. 9-55

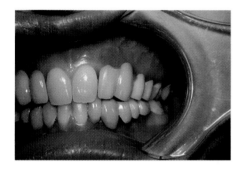

Fig. 9-56

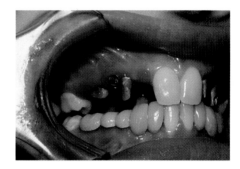

Fig. 9-57

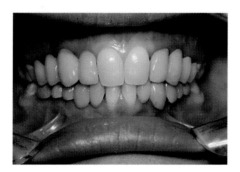

Fig. 9-58

Fixture loss rarely occurs after prosthetic completion. If a fixed implant prosthesis is involved and if the number of the remaining fixtures is inadequate for fixed support, the clinician must decide whether to convert permanently to an overdenture or to use an interim overdenture while healing occurs (additional implants can be placed in preparation for making a new fixed prosthesis). When fixture loss has occurred and inadequate fixtures remain to support the fixed prosthesis, either an existing complete denture can be modified or a new prosthesis can be made. If it is available, the old denture is relieved, and a tissue-conditioning material is used to reline the denture while healing occurs. When healing has occurred, attachments may be added to the denture.

10

Hygiene/Maintenance Guidelines

DEBORAH L. STEELE, R.D.H., B.S.
GAYLE S. ORTON, R.D.H., B.S., M.Ed.

Diligent and precise surgical and prosthetic procedures are critical to the success of implant therapy, but maintenance of implants may be of equal importance in ensuring a long-term, favorable prognosis. The dental professional's responsibility in providing supportive therapy and education in maintaining dental implants is crucial. This chapter will begin to define the clinician's responsibilities in examining and assessing the tissues surrounding the transmucosal abutment, as well as the implant fixture and its supporting prosthesis. Suggestions for the removal of hard and soft deposits, recommendations for home care procedures, and guidelines for appropriate professional maintenance intervals are included.

Examination of the Peri-implant Tissues and Prosthesis

Examination and assessment of the soft tissues surrounding the dental implant abutment and prosthesis provide the clinician with valuable information that may influence treatment planning. For example, the presence of hard and soft deposits and the current status of the peri-implant tissues will influence the kind and type of clinical procedures that need to be performed and the type of individualized home care instructions that must be offered.

Clinical assessment of peri-implant soft tissues begins with a visual examination. Characteristics of the soft tissue, including tone, color, contour, size, and consistency should be noted and compared to baseline records. The presence of inflamed or exuberant tissues should be documented and correlated with the presence of hard and soft deposits. Various maintenance record forms may be used for this purpose (Fig. 10-1). Clinicians may find it useful to record the presence or absence of keratinized tissues immediately surrounding the transmucosal abutment. As long as good oral hygiene levels are maintained, tissue health is probably not dependent on the existence of keratinized tissues. However, nonkeratinized tissue surrounding abutments may create a condition that is sensitive to the patient, influencing his or her ability to keep the abutment cylinders free of deposits.

The issue of routine probing for clinical assessment of the peri-implant tissues is currently being debated. Baseline probe readings may be recorded at the time of prosthesis delivery and before the appliance is seated. Thereafter, in the absence of pain, discomfort, or other clinical signs of disease (inflamed or exuberant tissues, mobility, or bone loss), the value of probing may be questioned. Appropriate clinical

Brånemark system®
Maintenance record

Patient's name _____

Chart # _____   Referring Dr. _____   Alternate recalls Y / N

Medical alert	Maintenance interval	Next appointment

Charting code (cc)*

		Months 2	Minutes 30	1. _____
B-Bleeding	M-Mobility	3	45	2. _____
C-Calculus	N-Normal	4	60	3. _____
D-Discharge/suppuration	NK-Nonkeratinized			
E-Edematous, soft	P-Plaque	6	90	4. _____
F-Fibrous enlargement	R-Redness			
K-Keratinized	S-Sensitivity			

Special considerations: _____
_____
_____
_____
_____

Date _____
DDS√: Y /N   Fee: _____

Changes
Medical history   Y / N _____
Dental history   Y / N _____
EO/IO exam   Y / N _____
Radiographs: (type)

Procedures performed

Tissue assessment   Y / N
Prosthesis removed   Y / N
Calculus removed   Y / N
Coronal polish   Y / N

Home care instructions

Recommended: _____
_____
_____

Uses: _____
_____
_____

Patient compliance: good/poor

Comments: _____
_____
_____

Signature: _____

Probing depths (of natural teeth)

	1-8	1-7	1-6	1-5	1-4	1-3	1-2	1-1	2-1	2-2	2-3	2-4	2-5	2-6	2-7	2-8
Fa																
*cc																
Li																
*cc																

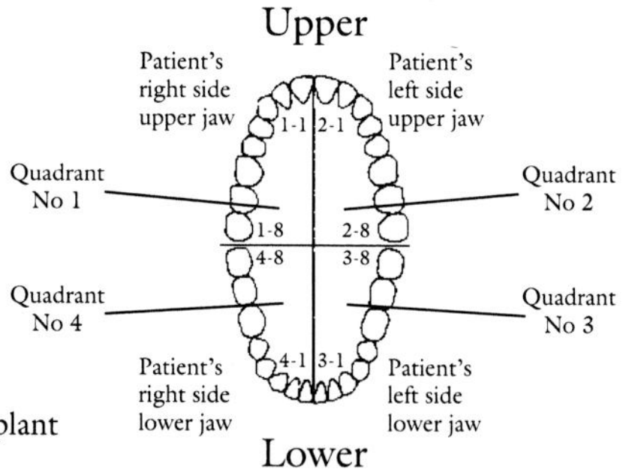

Upper

Patient's right side upper jaw
Patient's left side upper jaw
Quadrant No 1
Quadrant No 2
Quadrant No 4
Quadrant No 3
Patient's right side lower jaw
Patient's left side lower jaw

Lower

Designate implant abutment site in blue

	4-8	4-7	4-6	4-5	4-4	4-3	4-2	4-1	3-1	3-2	3-3	3-4	3-5	3-6	3-7	3-8
Li																
*cc																
Fa																
*cc																

Fig. 10-1

Date
DDS√: Y / N   Fee: _____

Changes
Medical history Y / N _____
Dental history   Y / N _____
EO/IO exam   Y / N _____
Radiographs: (type)

Procedures performed
Tissue assessment   Y / N
Prosthesis removed Y / N
Calculus removed   Y / N
Coronal polish   Y / N

Home care instructions

Recommended: _____
_____
_____
Uses: _____
_____

Patient compliance: good/poor

Comments: _____
_____
_____

Signature: _____

Probing Depths (of natural teeth)

	1-8	1-7	1-6	1-5	1-4	1-3	1-2	1-1	2-1	2-2	2-3	2-4	2-5	2-6	2-7	2-8
Fa																
*cc																
Li																
*cc																

Upper

Patient's right side upper jaw   Patient's left side upper jaw

Quadrant No 1   Quadrant No 2

1-8   2-8
4-8   3-8

Quadrant No 4   Quadrant No 3

Patient's right side lower jaw   Patient's left side lower jaw

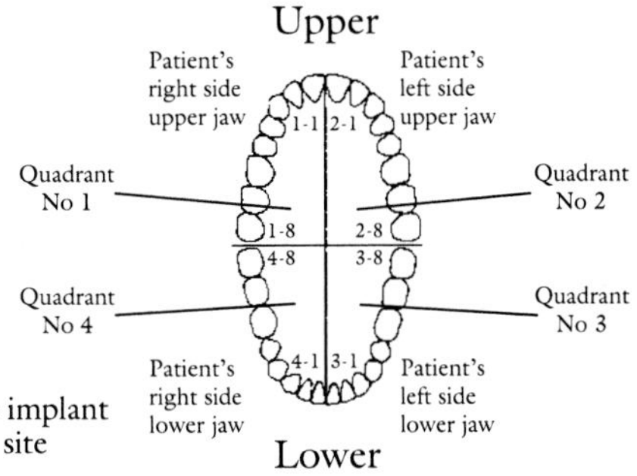

Designate implant abutment site in blue

Lower

	4-8	4-7	4-6	4-5	4-4	4-3	4-2	4-1	3-1	3-2	3-3	3-4	3-5	3-6	3-7	3-8
Li																
*cc																
Fa																
*cc																

Date _____
DDS√: Y /N   Fee: _____

Changes
Medical history Y / N _____
Dental history   Y / N _____
EO/IO exam   Y / N _____
Radiographs: (type)

Procedures performed

Tissue assessment   Y / N
Prosthesis removed   Y / N
Calculus removed   Y / N
Coronal polish   Y / N

Home care instructions

Recommended: _____
_____
_____
Uses: _____
_____

Patient compliance: good/poor

Comments: _____
_____
_____

Signature: _____

Probing Depths (of natural teeth)

	1-8	1-7	1-6	1-5	1-4	1-3	1-2	1-1	2-1	2-2	2-3	2-4	2-5	2-6	2-7	2-8
Fa																
*cc																
Li																
*cc																

Upper

Patient's right side upper jaw   Patient's left side upper jaw

Quadrant No 1   Quadrant No 2

1-8   2-8
4-8   3-8

Quadrant No 4   Quadrant No 3

Patient's right side lower jaw   Patient's left side lower jaw

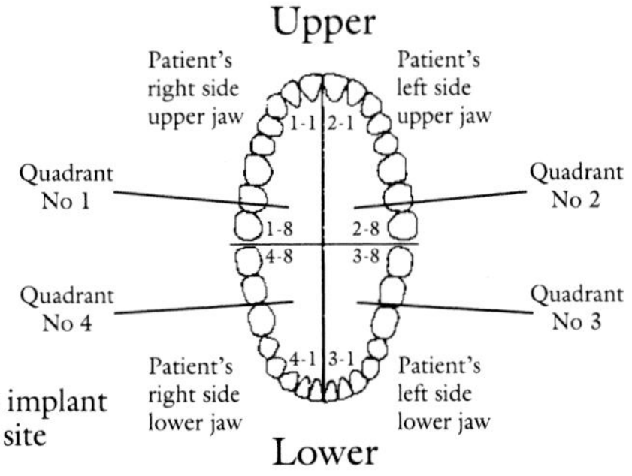

Designate implant abutment site in blue

Lower

	4-8	4-7	4-6	4-5	4-4	4-3	4-2	4-1	3-1	3-2	3-3	3-4	3-5	3-6	3-7	3-8
Li																
*cc																
Fa																
*cc																

Fig. 10-1—cont'd

judgment must be used in determining the need for probing. In any case, probing of the sulcus, if performed, must be atraumatic. If multiple abutments are connected by a prosthetic suprastructure, obtaining accurate probe readings may be difficult because of access problems in positioning the probe tip parallel to the long axis of the transmucosal abutment. Flexible plastic probes may reduce this problem; however the most accurate readings are obtained when the suprastructure is removed.

Absolute probe readings and attachment levels are not as critical in terms of the success or failure of an implant as are progressive changes in either of these two parameters over time. The average depth of the peri-implant sulcus varies because of a number of factors. Examples include abutment height, depth of fixture countersinking at Stage 1 surgery, and the amount of tissue thinning during Stage 2 surgery procedures. There may be instances in which the probing depth is greater than 4 mm and yet is still associated with a healthy, stable implant. Thicker fibrotic tissues, such as those located in the palatal region, provide a good example.

After the soft tissue has been assessed and documented, the presence or absence of mobility of the implant fixtures, the transmucosal abutments, and the prosthetic suprastructure should be evaluated. Many clinicians routinely remove the prosthesis yearly to definitively test for fixture and abutment mobility; others remove the suprastructure only if clinical signs and symptoms warrant the procedure. Since a successful osseointegrated implant has no periodontal ligament, zero mobility is anticipated around stable fixtures.

The absence of a periodontal ligament precludes the ability of the implant fixture to absorb any excess loading. Occlusal trauma of any magnitude from the prosthesis will negatively influence the surrounding supporting structures of the fixture and may lead to their destruction. If any mobility is present, optimal occlusion cannot be obtained. To check for mobility of the suprastructure, two instrument handles or the thumb and index finger of one hand can be used to attempt to physically move the prosthesis (Fig. 10-2). The clinician should be alert for the presence of salivary percolation at the interface where the prosthesis meets the coronal portion of the abutment cylinder. Small bubbles of saliva usually indicate a loose suprastructure. This necessitates a separate procedure in which the attending dentist removes the prosthesis, checks the gold screws for breakage, or determines the need for screw tightening. Mobility of a prosthesis that closely approximates the gingival tissues can only be determined by observing whether the prosthesis rocks when lateral pressure is applied.

Accurate assessment of transmucosal abutment mobility can only be performed if the suprastructure is removed (Fig. 10-3). If any movement of the transmucosal abutment is detected, the center abutment screw should be checked for the presence of a fracture. If none is found, a tightening of the center screw by the attending dentist may be all that is required.

Percussive testing of the transmucosal abutment has not been widely used as a peri-implant parameter to date. Clinicians who use percussion find that it is a helpful tool in assessing the presence or absence of sensitivity of the bone surrounding the fixture. Under optimal conditions, there should be no bone sensitivity during percussive testing. If sensitivity is found, it should be documented and correlated with other clinical findings.

Of all the clinical parameters used to assess the status of the dental implant, assessment of implant mobility and radiographic evaluation of the surrounding bone-implant interface currently remain the traditional modes of evaluation in determining the status of the osseointegrated fixture. Radiographs are useful in assessing bone height and density and in showing the functional relationship between the fixture, the abutment, and the prosthesis. Although it is a late sign, radiographic evidence of bone loss is the most reliable of all the conventional periodontal indices for evaluating fail-

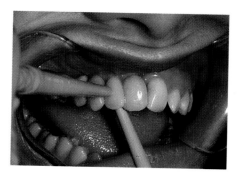

Fig. 10-2

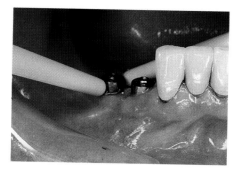

Fig. 10-3

ing implants. A failing and mobile fixture may display a thin radiolucent line at its bone interface.

Panoramic or periapical (perifixtural) baseline radiographs are taken at the time of the abutment connection procedure to ensure that the abutment has been seated properly on the fixture. A precise fit between the fixture head and abutment should be evident, with no intervening gap between the two. Perifixtural radiographs are taken subsequent to the seating of the prosthesis. Two views of each fixture are usually required to ensure a more accurate measurement of the marginal bone height around the fixture threads. Films are used as a baseline for comparison of bone height with future radiographs. If no film grid is used, bone loss may be assessed by comparing baseline bone height levels and by counting the number of fixture threads coronal to the bony crest. With the Nobelpharma fixture, the distance between each thread is 0.6 mm. An exact paralleling technique, as well as a standard kilovoltage, will improve radiographic diagnosis.

Protocols for radiographic intervals include baseline films when the prosthesis is seated and follow-up radiographs at 6 months, 1 year, and 3 years, following prosthesis insertion. Thereafter, radiographs are taken at 3-year intervals or as needed for necessary evaluation. Many clinicians rely on clinical signs of disease activity (inflammation, mobility, suppuration, recent history of bone loss, etc.) or symptoms, such as pain, sensitivity, or discomfort, to determine the need for additional radiographs.

Instrumentation

Calculus removal is accomplished by using a plastic scaler to avoid altering the metal surface (Figs. 10-4 through 10-7). Metal instruments, including ultrasonic scalers, are not recommended. Calculus that forms on the transmucosal abutments is primarily supragingival and can be similar to calculus forming on a natural tooth. It will sometimes *flake off* or easily fracture in large pieces. At other times, the calculus is fine in nature, and its adherence to the abutment cylinder can be tenacious (Fig. 10-8). When it is dried with air, thin calculus may take on a burnished, dull, or translucent appearance.

A major goal of transmucosal abutment instrumentation is to avoid roughening the surface. A roughened surface may promote subsequent bacterial plaque accumulation and calculus formation. Additionally, surface alteration of the tin oxide layer has the potential to affect the biological properties of the surface. Whether a roughened surface has an adverse effect on cell attachment to titanium has not been firmly established in the scientific literature; however, this may be an important consideration.

Following the removal of hard deposits, the prosthesis and transmucosal abutments may be selectively polished with a rubber cup, rubber prophy point, and tufted floss or flossing cord (Figs. 10-9 through 10-11). Aluminum oxide polishing paste is recommended to avoid unnecessary scratching of the titanium abutments and the prosthetic suprastructure. Stains on the suprastructure may require a medium grit abrasive for complete stain removal.

Patient Education

The long-term success of the dental implant lies, to a great extent, in the ability of the patient to control daily plaque accumulation. The dental professional plays an important role in assisting and influencing the dental patient to maintain adequate oral hygiene levels. The challenge to the dental patient may be one of access, for it is often difficult to physically reach all areas of the supragingival appliance despite high levels of motivation. On the other hand, many patients exhibit low dental IQs, as evidenced by their denture history. These individuals often require special consideration and patience on the part of the dental professional. More frequent recall intervals may be necessary to encourage compliance. Home care instructions should be reviewed and reinforced at each appointment. Written instructions are often helpful. A variety of cleaning methods may be recommended, depending on the type of design of the prosthesis.

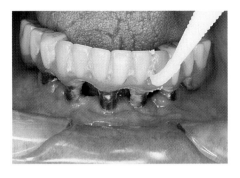

Fig. 10-4

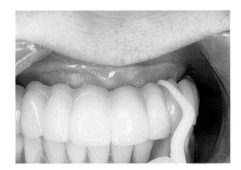

Fig. 10-5

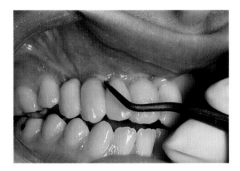

Fig. 10-6

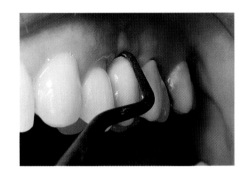

Fig. 10-7

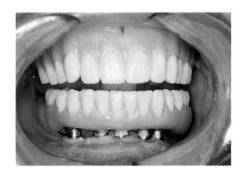

Fig. 10-8

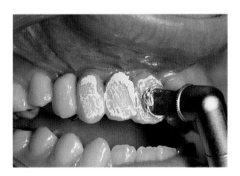

Fig. 10-9

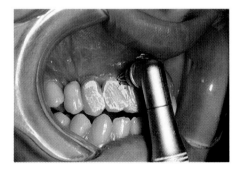

Fig. 10-10

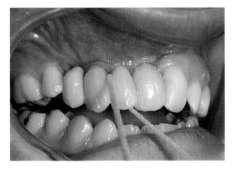

Fig. 10-11

Recommendations after Phase 2 Surgery

Absence of microbiota is essential for tissue healing; therefore, the presence of plaque will retard the healing process. After the periodontal pack has been removed, plaque forms readily on the abutments.

Initial oral hygiene instructions are given at the time of periodontal pack and suture removal. Recommendations include rinsing with salt water twice a day, until the tissue swelling subsides. A twice daily, 30-second chlorhexidine (Peridex) rinse is recommended for at least 1 week following Stage 2 surgery. In some cases rinsing may be continued until the final prosthesis is seated; this is at the clinician's discretion. A soft toothbrush or flat end-tuft brush is used in addition to rinsing (Fig. 10-12). Gentle brushing is important because the patient may experience soft tissue sensitivity for a period of time following the surgical procedure.

Recommendations for Complete and Partially Edentulous Patients

An assortment of brushes may be used to effectively remove soft deposits. A standard toothbrush is usually recommended for the facial, lingual, and occlusal surfaces of the prosthetic suprastructure. A nylon-coated interdental brush is effective for plaque removal on the gingival side of the suprastructure and proximal surfaces of the abutments. A flat end-tuft brush is indicated on the facial surfaces of the abutment cylinders. This brush is angled at 45 degrees toward the gingival tissues and moved in a circular, vibratory motion. The tapered end-tuft brush is preferred for plaque removal on lingual abutment surfaces. The brush head may be bent to improve access to this area (Fig. 10-13).

Prosthetic bridge design and patient dexterity dictate selection of the type of floss or flossing cord. A flossing cord specifically designed for dental implants, *polishes* the transmucosal abutments and the gingival side of the prosthesis. The hooked end of the cord is used as a threading device, making insertion between adjacent abutment cylinders relatively easy (Fig. 10-14). Once inserted, the cord is *crisscrossed* and moved from side to side and up and down to reach the entire circumference of the abutment (Fig. 10-15). A thinner cord for tight embrasures may be used; the cord is durable enough to be used several times by simply rinsing and drying after each use.

Rotary brushes may be a helpful adjunct to the home care regimen. Caution should be taken in areas of nonkeratinized tissue or fixture thread exposure (Fig. 10-16).

Recommendations for Single Tooth Prosthesis

Home care recommendations for cleaning the single tooth implant prosthesis vary, depending on the prosthetic and abutment design and on its location in the mouth. A soft toothbrush is recommended for brushing the crown and prosthetic components surrounded by the gingiva. If the transmucosal abutment is placed subgingivally, regular dental floss or tufted floss may be used. The prosthetic tooth is flossed in the same manner as a natural tooth, wrapping the floss around the narrow circumference of the abutment cylinder (Fig. 10-17). Nylon-coated interdental brushes are helpful in cleaning the proximal surfaces. The appropriate brush size is determined by the space available, which varies greatly from patient to patient.

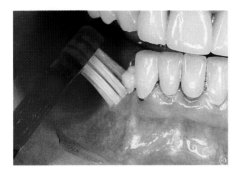

Fig. 10-12

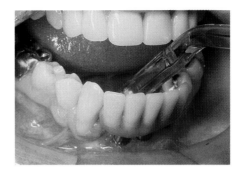

Fig. 10-13

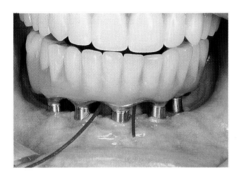

Fig. 10-14

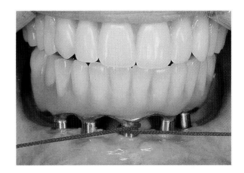

Fig. 10-15

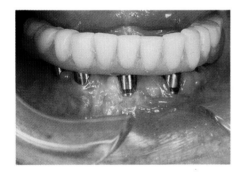

Fig. 10-16

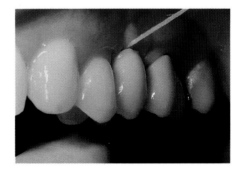

Fig. 10-17

Recommendations for Overdenture Prosthesis

Home care for the patient with an overdenture is facilitated by removing the overdenture. The transmucosal abutments may be brushed with either a standard soft toothbrush or a flat end-tuft brush (Fig. 10-18). If the abutment cylinders are connected with a bar, floss or a flossing cord is easily inserted under the bar and then wrapped around each abutment cylinder for cleaning (Fig. 10-19).

Cleaning the undersurface of the prosthesis, the overdenture framework, and the proximal surfaces of the abutment cylinders may be accomplished by using a nylon-coated interdental brush (Fig. 10-20). Patients should be encouraged to replace the interdental brushes frequently because the underlying metal wire, if exposed, may scratch the titanium surface.

A daily soaking of the overdenture in a commercial cleaning solution is recommended. If no metal is present on the prosthesis, an overnight soaking in full-strength white vinegar once each week is helpful in removing stubborn stains.

At the clinician's discretion, other adjunctive oral hygiene aids, such as rubber tips and wooden picks, may be recommended. A toothpaste accepted by the American Dental Association may be used during brushing. Twice daily antimicrobial rinses, such as chlorhexidine, may be beneficial if patients are unable to maintain adequate oral hygiene levels. These individuals should be informed of possible side effects, such as staining and taste alteration. Altered taste may be minimized by using the rinse at least 1 hour after food consumption.

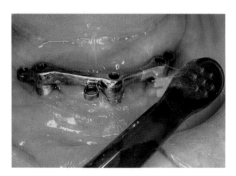
Fig. 10-18

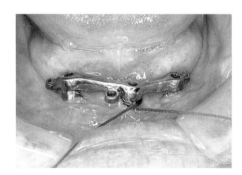
Fig. 10-19

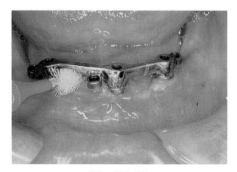
Fig. 10-20

Subgingival oral irrigation may be a helpful adjunct for selected patients. Caution must be taken to adjust the rate of flow to the lowest setting. The patient is instructed to direct the antimicrobial solution into the sulcus, allowing the solution to gently flood the sulcus.

Other home care recommendations and instructions are influenced by the location, angulation, and length of the transmucosal abutments; the prosthetic design; the patient's oral habits, motivation, manual dexterity, and oral health. Careful, individualized instruction is usually required with any dental implant patient.

Maintenance Intervals

Maintenance intervals are determined by a number of factors, such as the amount of plaque and calculus formation, the condition of the soft tissues, the status of the prosthesis, the patient's commitment to meticulous home care, and various health considerations of the patient. Appropriate recall intervals are determined on an individual basis, taking into consideration the patient's history and present evaluation.

A suggested time frame may be the following:

1. At prosthesis delivery
    * Comprehensive oral hygiene instructions
    * Baseline data documented
2. One month following prosthesis delivery
    * Review of home care techniques
    * Calculus removal and coronal polish, if needed
3. Three months later
    * Examination of tissues
    * Calculus removal and coronal polish, if needed
    * Home care reinforcement
    * Establish recall interval (between 3 and 6 months, determined by the history and current assessment)

11

Implant Systems

Successful, sound research by the Swedish team created an osseointegrated implant that can have a predictable and reliable prognosis for clinical treatment. Because of the knowledge and experience gained through the Branemark system, other implant systems have used this research to develop and market endosseous implant systems. Some of the systems should be discussed, although research for comparing all the systems simultaneously is limited.

The following implant systems (other than the Branemark system) are the systems in which this team has had direct case study and application either in clinical/laboratory, or laboratory only. We recognize the vast numbers of systems in the industry, but we are mentioning only the following ones because they are the most widely used at this time.

Calcitek (Integral Corp.)

The Calcitek implant system was developed as a hydroxylapatite (HA) bone substitute in 1981. The company's synthetic polycrystalline ceramic hydroxylapatite, Calcitite HA, is completely biocompatible and essentially nonresorbable. It is a two-stage surgery system performed by an oral surgeon.

The Calcitek/Integral system offers a variety of fixture implants in a range of sizes. The Integral fixture is available in a 3.25 mm and 4.0 mm diameter at 8 mm, 10 mm, 13 mm, and 15 mm lengths. The Integral Omniloc (antirotational) fixture is available in the above-mentioned diameters and lengths, with the addition of an 18 mm length.

The prosthetic components for the fixtures include fixed, preangled, shouldered, and wide-base shouldered abutments; impression post abutment; analogue coping screw; waxing sleeve; waxing post; and overdenture attachments. There are option components for each fixture discussed.

Dentsply/Spectra-System (Formerly Core-Vent)

The Dentsply/Spectrum System (Core-Vent) that was developed by Dr. Gerald Niznick (1984, 1985, and 1986) offers a variety of component fixture sizes and designs for different treatment planning. This system uses a two-stage surgical technique that does not require an oral surgeon to place the implanted fixture. The implants are either screw-type designs with perforations or hollow-basket design. The fixture name—Core-Vent, Screw-Vent, Micro-Vent, and Bio-Vent—is descriptive of the design available for the treatment plan selection.

The implant fixture is made of a titanium alloy (90% titanium, 6% aluminum, and 4% vanadium) and is available in 3.5 mm and 4.5 mm diameter, either threaded or beveled hex-threaded, in 8 mm, 10.5 mm, 13 mm, and 16 mm lengths. It also comes in a 5.5 mm diameter, with a hex-hole, and in the same lengths that were previously described. The threaded screw design fixture has a horizontal and a vertical vent at the apex. It is made of commercially pure titanium and is available in 3.75 mm diameter with either threaded or hex-hole in 7 mm, 10 mm, 13 mm, or 16 mm lengths.

The prosthetic components for the fixtures include a hex-lock abutment, angled titanium abutment, titanium-threaded inserts, plastic-castable coping insets, plastic-castable inserts for threaded implants, titanium coping inserts, titanium nonbendable inserts, overdenture attachments, and resilient attachments. The numerous prosthetic components are specific for each system discussed.

IMZ System

The Interpore IMZ system requires a two-stage surgical technique. Initial development and work on this implant system were done in West Germany by Axel Kirsch, D.D.S. (1980 and 1983), and it has been in clinical use since 1978. The non-threaded implant is made from commercially pure titanium, and the surface is spray-coated with plasma to increase surface areas sixfold for bone interface. The IMZ implant is available in 3.3 mm diameter, with 8 mm, 10 mm, 13 mm, and 15 mm lengths, and 4.0 mm diameter, with 8 mm, 11 mm, 13 mm, and 15 mm lengths. The smaller diameter implant is advantageous in severely resorbed bone with narrow buccolingual width.

The prosthetic components for the fixtures include an intramobile element (IME) and a transmucossal implant extension (TIE). This system can be used for either edentulous or partially edentulous patients.

◆ STERI-OSS SYSTEM

The Steri-Oss system (Denar Corporation) uses a two-stage surgical technique. The implant is made from 99.5% pure titanium and offers a tapered apex thread design, and the coronal third includes a periodontal neck. When bone loss occurs, the long, highly polished neck of the fixture is exposed, instead of a threaded surface like other implant systems.

The implant fixture is available in a 3.5 mm and a 4.0 mm diameter in 12 mm, 16 mm, and 20 mm lengths, as well as in a miniseries. The miniseries is available in 3.8 mm diameter in 8 mm, 10 mm, and 12 mm lengths. It has a shorter polished neck surface and a longer threaded area with increased number of threads per millimeter.

The prosthetic components for the fixtures are interchangeable because of the uniform abutment threading for all sizes of implants. Attachments include the coventional coronal screw, telescoping abutment, magnetic attachment, O-ring attachment, and several abutments for direct cementation.[11]

BIBLIOGRAPHY

1. Adell R, Kekholm U, Rockle B, Branemark PI: A 15-year study of osseointegrated implants in the treatment of the edentulous jaw, *Int J Oral Surg* 10:387-416, 1981.
2. Albrektsson T, Branemark PI, Hansson HA, Lindstrom J: Osseointegrated titanium implant: requirements for ensuring a long-lasting, direct, bone-to-implant anchorage in man, *ACTA Orthop Scand* 52:155-170, 1981.
3. Albrektsson T, Zarb G: *The Branemark osseointegrated implant,* Lombard, Ill, 1989, Quintessence.
4. Blustein R et al: *Int J Oral Maxillofac Implants* 1:47-49, 1986.
5. Branemark PI et al: *Osseointegrated implants in the treatment of the edentulous jaw: experience from a 10-year period,* Stockholm, Sweden, 1977, Almqvist & Wiksell International.
6. Branemark PI, Zarb G, Albrektsson T: *Tissue integrated prosthesis: osseointegration in clinical dentistry,* Lombard, Ill, 1985, Quintessence.
7. Dahlin C et al: Generation of new bone around titanium implants using a membrane technique: an experimental study in rabbits, 4:14-25, 1989.
8. Eriksson AR, Albrektsson T: Temperature threshold for heat-induced bone injury: a vital-microscopic study in the rabbit, *J Prosthet Dent* 50(1), 1983.
9. Fredrickson E, Gress M: Laboratory procedures for osseointegrated implants, *QDT Yearbook* 12:15-37, 1988.
10. Frost H: Vital biomechanics: proposed general concepts for skeletal adaptations to mechanical usage, *Calcif Tissue Int* 42:145-156, 1988.
11. Hobo S, Ichida E, Garcia L: *Osseointegration and occlusal rehabilitation: osseointegration implant systems,* 2:23-29, 1989.
12. Kahnberg KE, Nystrom E, Bartholdsson L: Combined use of bone grafts and Branemark fixtures in the treatment of severely resorbed maxillae, *Int J Oral Maxillofac Implants* 4:297-304, 1989.
13. Klinge B, Petersson A, Maly P: Location of the mandibular canal: comparison of microscopic findings, conventional radiography, and computed tomography, *Int J Oral Maxillofac Implants* 4:327-332, 1989.
14. Lekholm U: Clinical procedures for treatment with osseointegrated dental implants, *J Prosthet Dent* 50(1), 1983.
15. Lindquist L, Rockler B, Carlsson G: Bone resorption around fixtures in edentulous patients treated with mandibular fixed tissue-integrated prostheses, *J Prosthet Dent* 59(2), 1988.
16. Listrom R, Symington J: Osseointegrated dental implants in conjunction with bone grafts, *Int J Oral Maxillofac Surg* 17:116-118, 1988.
17. Nyman S, Lang N, Buser D, Bragger U: Bone regeneration adjacent to titanium dental implants using guided tissue regeneration, *Int J Oral Maxillofac Implants* 5:9-14, 1990.
18. Parel S, Sullivan D: *Esthetics and osseointegration,* Dallas, 1989, Taylor.
19. Schwarz M, Rothman S, Rhodes M, Chafetz N: Computed tomography. Part 1. Preoperative assessment of the mandible for endosseous implant surgery, *Int J Oral Maxillofac Implants* 2:137-141, 1987.
20. Schwarz M, Rothman S, Rhodes M, Chafetz N: Computed tomography. Part 2. Preoperative assessment of the mandible for endosseous implant surgery, *Int J Oral Maxillofac Implants* 2:143-148, 1987.
21. Wook R, Moore D: Grafting of the maxillary sinus with intraorally harvested autogenous bone prior to implant placement, *Int J Oral Maxillofac Implants* 3:209-214, 1988.
22. Worthington P, Bolender C, Taylor T: The Swedish system of osseointegrated implants: problems and complications encountered during a 4-year trial period, *Int J Oral Maxillofac Implants* 2:77-84, 1987.

SUGGESTED READINGS

Adell R et al: Marginal tissue reactions at osseointegrated titanium fixtures: a 3-year longitudinal prospective study, *Int J Oral Maxillofac Surg* 15:39-52, 1986.

Dmytryk J, Fox S, Moriarty J: The effects of scaling titanium implant surfaces with metal and plastic instruments on cell attachment, *J Periodont* 61:491-496, 1990.

Fox S, Moriarty J, Kusy R: The effects of scaling a titanium implant surface with metal and plastic instruments: an in vitro study, *J Periodont* 61:485-490, 1990.

Lekholm U et al: Marginal tissue reactions at osseointegrated titanium fixtures (11): a cross-sectional retrospective study, *Int J Oral Maxillofac Surg* 15:53-61, 1986.

Orton G, Steele D, Wolinsky L: The dental professional's role in monitoring and maintenance of tissue-integrated prostheses, *Int J Oral Maxillofac Implants* 4:305-310, 1989.

Rapley J, Swan R et al: The surface characteristics produced by various oral hygiene instruments and materials on titanium implant abutments, *Int J Oral Maxillofac Implants* 5:47-52, 1990.

van Steenberghe D: Periodontal aspects of osseointegrated oral implants ad modum Branemark, *Dent Clin North Am* 32:355-370, 1988.

ACKNOWLEDGMENTS

Documentation photos from:

1. Richard Roccanova, Spokane Washington; Gary Maxwell, Spokane Washington:, *CeraOne single tooth metal restoration.*
2. Kenji Higuchi: *Surgical procedures.*
3. Nobelpharma Industries: *Educational information/documentation of CeraOne abutment.*
4. Edward Fredrickson, Patrick Stevens, Spokane, Washington; James Clark, Lewiston, Idaho: *Hygiene/maintenance guidelines.*
5. William LaVelle, Iowa City, Iowa: *Cleft palate rehabilitation.*
6. Anne Fyler, Iowa City, Iowa: *Auricular prosthesis.*

Index

*Page numbers in *italics* indicate illustrations.

178